ADHD IS NOT A FOUR LETTER WORD

Copyright © 2014 by Karen Ryan
First Edition – May 2014

ISBN
978-1-4602-3932-2 (Hardcover)
978-1-4602-3933-9 (Paperback)
978-1-4602-3934-6 (eBook)

I would like to thank those who believed in me and helped me along the way .... namely my husband, Ed, my son, Eddy, my daughter, Jessica, my two sisters Gabriella and Deborah, and my good friend Teresa Vaccaro.

Disclaimer: The material in this book is for informational purposes only. Every person has a unique and individual situation and therefore should seek advice from a healthcare professional before undertaking major changes in diet, exercise, etc. The author and publisher expressly disclaim responsibility for any adverse effects resulting from the use or application of the information contained in this book.

Produced by:

FriesenPress
Suite 300 – 852 Fort Street
Victoria, BC, Canada V8W 1H8

www.friesenpress.com

Distributed to the trade by The Ingram Book Company

For my family . . .
Always.

ADHD IS NOT A FOUR LETTER WORD

*Drug-Free Strategies for Managing
the Gift That Is ADHD*

· · · · · · · · · · · · · · · · ·

Karen Ryan

Table of Contents

Educate before you medicate!
—Unknown

INTRODUCTION

In the last two decades, Attention Deficit Hyperactivity Disorder, or ADHD, has increased by 20 percent and scientists are striving to find out why. What has changed in our lives to cause these numbers to explode? Is it the environment—the air we breathe, the water we drink, the food we eat? Starting from the moment we are conceived, nutrients are absorbed from our own mothers. Whatever they put in their mouths comes directly to us . . . and it all starts there!

ADHD is not a new phenomenon; it has been around since the early 1700s, back when it was known as "Moral Imbecility" or "Post-Encephalitic Behaviour Disorder." Since that time, scientists and researchers have frantically been trying to figure out where, why, and what: Where did it come from? Why does it happen? What happened to the human brain to cause it?

Science has come a long way in answering some of these questions, but by doing so, new questions have cropped up. One of the most controversial of those questions is, "What is the best way to treat this disorder?" What was once considered a childhood disorder has emerged as a disorder afflicting the masses. People as old as sixty and up are being diagnosed with ADHD and, at the same time, are finding relief to know that 1) there is a name for it, 2) they are not alone, and 3) there is treatment, help, and support for them.

So let's go back to the original question: What is the best way to treat this disorder? There is really no easy answer to this somewhat complicated issue, as many people will tell you many different things. Go to your psychiatrist and he will say, "Medication!" Go to your family doctor and she will say, "Medication!" Ask your child's teacher and she too will say, "Medication!" But go to your naturopath, dietitian, or nutritionist, and all of these people will tell you what I'm about to tell you: "There is no *one* effective treatment for ADHD." ADHD is complex. Therefore, it requires a multi-pronged approach that consists of education, support at home, support at school, proper diet, vitamins and minerals, routine, patience, and, of course, love.

You may ask, "Why would I want to spend all this time and energy on a so-called 'multi-pronged approach' when I can just give my kid a pill and he's good for a few hours or sometimes even for the rest of the day?" True enough, you can do that. But what I bet you didn't know about, and what your child's psychiatrist, doctor, counsellor, or teacher didn't tell you, are the severe, sometimes deadly side effects and ramifications that come from these pills.

First of all, these ADHD medications—called methylphenidates—are considered Schedule II drugs. Street drugs are Schedule I narcotics. A little too close for comfort in my eyes. Second, these ADHD medications are classified by the FDA and Health Canada as being in the same family as cocaine and speed. So, knowing that, here's some food for thought: Would you give your six- or seven-year-old child two lines of cocaine in the morning before school, and then ask his teacher to ensure that he has two more lines at lunchtime? I thought not. Then why would you give your child a pill that exhibits the exact same effects and side effects as a Schedule I narcotic?

If you're thinking that this a gross exaggeration, then you're mistaken. These pills don't have minor side effects; they have major ones, including ticks, loss of appetite, trouble sleeping, stomach pains, suicidal thoughts, increased heart rate, nausea, psychosis, seizures, respiratory problems, heart problems, sudden death . . . Shall I go on? The mere fact that methylphenidates even bear a structural relationship to cocaine should give some serious pause for thought.

The point I'm trying to get across is this: ADHD medication is not to be taken lightly. What I'm truly hoping is that you will at least exhaust all other avenues before venturing into the world of medication, because once you go there, it's a whole new ball game.

I want to tell you a little story about why I am such a huge advocate for this and why I vehemently believe that it's not acceptable to be giving children—or anyone, for that matter—ADHD medication, whether it is of the stimulant or the non-stimulant variety. I would really like for you to put yourself in my shoes while reading this, if only for a minute . . .

Back in 2006, at the age of seven, my son was diagnosed with ADHD. My husband and I were not really surprised by the diagnosis. We knew by the time he was three that he probably had it, but decided not to act on it until it started to affect his schoolwork. My son's preschool teacher, kindergarten teacher, and first grade teacher all had asked me to have him tested, but I refused purely on the basis that, at the time, it wasn't affecting his schoolwork or his academic ability to learn. Then the second grade came along, and his teacher sat me down for a heart-to-heart chat and admitted that it was affecting not only his schoolwork but also the schoolwork of his classmates. Because she was professional about it and sincerely wanted my son to succeed without putting a label on him, we agreed to have him tested.

After many appointments at the mental health department of a children's hospital, a final diagnosis was made. Sure enough, my son did, in fact, have ADHD. The doctor's suggestion?

Medication, of course. At the time, we thought, "Well, if you can't trust your doctor, then who can you trust?" So we agreed to try the medication.

The first attempt was with Concerta. This worked somewhat, but once his body got used to it, it no longer worked properly. It was also much too difficult to regulate, as it jumps in nine to fifteen milligram increments, which was far too large for my liking. My son experienced a multitude of side effects that included trouble sleeping, stomach pains, dry mouth, internal twitching, loss of appetite, and an overall sense of "I feel weird!" Additionally, he was growing so fast that his doctor kept wanting to increase the dosage, and we were not entirely comfortable with this either. Her suggestion? Let's try Adderall! Our son was still only seven years old at this time, but again, trusting his doctor, we agreed to it. It was evident after the first few hours that this medication was not going to work out, as it just sucked the life right out of him—the spunk was gone, the energy was gone . . . Our son was gone. He experienced the same side effects as with Concerta, but the biggest one was that he was almost comatose; he literally would sit and stare into space for long periods of time. Even his teacher agreed that he was definitely not the same person. So I set up an appointment with his doctor relatively quickly, and her suggestion was—you guessed it—another medication! This time, however, it was a non-stimulant drug called Strattera. This is the part where things get scary.

Unlike Concerta and Adderall, which work very quickly, Strattera takes about four to six weeks to kick in before you can notice anything. After the four-week mark, we noticed that it had similar effects to Concerta, except the side effects were worse.

About five weeks after my son started treatment, I woke up one night around midnight. What woke me up was the fact that our house was freezing. I just assumed that the cat had somehow managed to push the front door open, so I checked both the front and back doors. Both were shut and locked tight. Next I checked the basement door. Everything was fine there too. So lastly, I decided to check the kids' rooms, which were upstairs. What I walked into would break any parent's heart.

My daughter's room was fine, as was my daughter, but my son had his window wide open and was sitting on the edge of his bed. I asked him quietly, "Hey, buddy, how are you doing? Is everything okay? Why is your window open?" He replied with six powerful words that forever changed my life: "I don't want to live anymore!" He didn't know why; he just did not want to exist on this earth any longer. I had a seven-year-old son who was suicidal—not because of mental illness or a scary movie he had watched, but because of the medication. I won't go into detail about the rest, but what I will tell you is that when I phoned his psychiatrist the next morning, her response was, "Wow, okay, let's take him off this medication immediately, and we'll get him started on something different!" My response? "Thanks, but your services are no longer needed!" And that was it. The ball was then officially in my court, and *I* was going to deal with it.

I have an extensive background in nutrition working for several health authorities as well as working as a nutrition counsellor one-on-one for various dietary needs. After this episode with my son, I decided to drop everything I was doing and have spent the last seven years researching ADHD, intensely focusing on everything from nutrition and supplements, to exercise, to ADHD coaching and counselling, and so on. I have made it my life's passion and breathe it, eat it, speak it, preach it, coach it, and work with parents, teachers, coaches, adults, adolescents, and children on any non-medicinal strategies for dealing and living with ADHD. I understand why parents (and teachers) often desperately push for an ADHD diagnosis and so quickly want to administer that rescuing prescription. Yes, the drugs can sometimes have beneficial short-term effects, but the long-term effects haven't been determined. I have written this book directed at the parent who is living and struggling with a child or teen with ADHD, but note that most of the strategies involved can be used by adults who have ADHD as well.

I will never tell a parent, "Do not medicate your child!" But what I will tell them is this: Here is a book that will give you every strategy under the sun, other than medication, to help you cope. If you have exhausted every resource possible, then do what you have to do. Just please don't make ADHD medication your first choice!

These children are not disordered.
They may have a different style of thinking, attending, and behaving,
but it's the broader social and educational influences
that create the disorder, not the children. (sic)
—Thomas Armstrong, PhD

WHAT ADHD IS
(AND WHAT IT IS NOT)

If you're reading this book, then chances are that either you are living with someone who has ADHD or you have it yourself. Either way, I always feel that the "definition" of ADHD needs to be addressed up front, as there are so many false implications that go along with it. It is not the "four-letter word" that everyone thinks it is but, rather, a gift that people just don't understand how to use. For some reason, ADHD seems to have a bad rap; it is consistently viewed as a negative "disorder" rather than as a positive attribute. To be honest, if I were coaching any sports team, I would hope that more than half of the kids on the team would have ADHD, as they are far more spunky, energetic, and creative.

ADHD is an acronym for Attention Deficit Hyperactivity Disorder, and believe it or not, it has been recognized since the early 1700s. It is characterized by significant difficulties of inattention, hyperactivity, and impulsiveness. Whereas ADHD used to be known simply as Attention Deficit Disorder, or ADD, it was renamed in 1994, as the problems with hyperactivity and impulsivity were not appropriately covered by the old term. Unfortunately, there is no blood test to determine whether or not someone has ADHD, so it is defined by symptoms rather than by cause.

The *DSM IV*, the *Diagnostic and Statistical Manual of Mental Disorders* (fourth edition), was published by the American Psychiatric Association in 1994 (the first edition being published in 1952) and is currently in its fifth edition. It establishes the criteria for the diagnosis of ADHD and lists symptoms that must appear before the age of seven. These symptoms must be present in two or more settings (i.e., home, school, work, or community) and for a time period of more than six months. The *DSM IV* is under constant scrutiny by many people, including psychiatrists, doctors, therapists, parents, and even its author. If anyone were to read its list of criteria that so matter-of-factly states, "Yes, you in fact do have ADHD!" then almost every individual in this nation would have this condition.

ADHD is broken down into three subtypes, each with its own pattern of behaviours:

ADHD Combined Type: This subtype occurs when both inattention and hyperactivity–impulsivity symptoms are present in an individual.

ADHD Predominantly Inattentive Type: This subtype occurs when there is inattention, but not enough hyperactivity-impulsivity symptoms are present. More often than not, girls are usually diagnosed with this subtype. This is because, as one myth states, girls have been socially conditioned to speak out less in class and be less disruptive.

ADHD Predominantly Hyperactive-Impulsive Type: This subtype occurs when there is hyperactivity and impulsivity, but not enough inattention symptoms are present.

ADHD is a condition that someone is born with or arises as a result of trauma to the neurology of the brain. It does not develop due to any of the following:

- poor diet
- bad parenting
- watching too much television
- playing too many video games
- bad schools
- socio-economic conditions
- eating too much sugar
- hormones

It also does not discriminate. No matter what your ethnic background is or what neighbourhood you live in, ADHD can happen to anyone. But there are a few things scientists are certain about regarding the causes of ADHD:

- ADHD is highly heritable (it is passed down predominantly from the father's side of the family but can come from the maternal line as well).
- Research has unveiled a strong correlation between ADHD and fetal alcohol syndrome.
- Environmental factors such as cigarette smoking and alcohol use during pregnancy can initiate ADHD.
- Brain injuries can prompt ADHD.
- Consumption of certain food additives—namely, artificial colours and preservatives—can trigger ADHD.

THE WORLD OF ADHD MEDICATION

I would like to touch on this subject, as I feel it is important to know what drugs are currently out on the market and what kinds of side effects go along with them. Many parents are oblivious to these side effects and do not want to believe that they occur. But they are very real, and children and adolescents throughout the world die from them every year. There are two main groups of ADHD drugs: stimulant medication and non-stimulant medication.

Stimulant Medication

Stimulant medication was introduced in the 1950s, having first been invented to treat narcolepsy, and is the most commonly used treatment for ADHD. While active in the human system, it can improve ADHD symptoms in about 70 percent of adults and 70 percent to 80 percent of children. It works by reducing interruptive behaviour, fidgeting, and other hyperactive symptoms, and also helps a person finish tasks and improve relationships. These effects sound great but, like many things in life, come at a price and are almost too good to be true.

Some stimulants have caused sudden death in children and adolescents with serious heart problems or congenital heart defects. Alarmingly, there is a growing popularity for college and university students to use these drugs even though they have not been diagnosed with ADHD. These students find that stimulant medication helps them study more effectively, stay awake longer, and focus better. This can result in serious problems, because sometimes, people are not aware of whether or not they have a heart condition, such as a murmur, and take the medication unknowingly. Additionally, scientific research now shows that there is a potential for abuse and addiction in the doses used to treat ADHD in children and adolescents.

Some of the most common stimulants include these prescription drugs:

- Ritalin
- Concerta
- Adderall and Adderall XR
- Vyvanse
- Biphentin
- Dexedrine
- Focalin and Focalin XR

While these are the most popular, there are many, many more on the market.

How Does Stimulant Medication Work?

Stimulant medication is fast-acting and generally will work within thirty minutes of consumption. It is also short-lasting and therefore will need to be taken up to three times per day.

The neurotransmitters present in ADHD are norepinephrine and dopamine, which either stimulate an area of brain cells or repress an area of brain cells. Simply speaking, for someone to be focused and able to pay attention, the brain cells must be stimulated. And for someone to be in control of impulsivity, the brain cells must be repressed. Stimulant medication does both. This, in turn, helps transmit signals between the nerves.

It is believed that in ADHD sufferers, the frontal lobe of the brain, also known as the "central processor," contains a reduced amount of norepinephrine and is thus responsible for the inability to focus and be attentive. Reduced dopamine fails to adequately repress the impulse actions. So, in plain terms, stimulant medication increases the levels of both norepinephrine and dopamine to boost functionality. But just as a reminder, remember that even though stimulant medication sometimes improves ADHD symptoms, that improvement comes at a price.

Side Effects Associated with Stimulant Medication

This is the easy part—there are more daunting side effects than there are positive ones. Here are just a few:

- loss of appetite
- increased heart rate, blood pressure, and body temperature
- dilation of pupils
- disturbed sleep patterns
- nausea
- bizarre, erratic, and sometimes violent behaviour
- hallucinations, hyperexcitability, and irritability
- panic
- convulsions, seizures, and death from high doses
- permanent damage to blood vessels of heart and brain; high blood pressure leading to heart attacks, strokes, and death
- liver, kidney, and lung damage
- destruction of tissues in nose if sniffed

- respiratory problems if smoked
- infectious diseases and abscesses if injected
- malnutrition and weight loss
- disorientation, apathy, and confused exhaustion
- strong psychological dependence
- psychosis
- depression
- damage to the brain, including strokes and possibly epilepsy
- suicidal thoughts
- suicide

No need to continue. I think you get the picture!

Non-Stimulant Medication and How It Works

Non-stimulant medication works differently than stimulant medication and is used in place of its counterpart, as stimulants are not often the "best fit." These drugs also increase the amount of norepinephrine in the brain and help ADHD by increasing attention span and reducing impulsive behaviour and hyperactivity. Like stimulant medication, non-stimulant medication does sometimes improve ADHD symptoms. But again, that improvement is laden with risks.

Non-stimulants have some advantages over many stimulants used to treat ADHD:

- They do not cause agitation or sleeplessness.
- They are not controlled substances and thus do not pose the same risk of abuse or addiction.
- They have a longer-lasting and smoother effect than many stimulants, which can wear off abruptly.

There are currently very few non-stimulant medications on the market for ADHD. The most widely used one today is Straterra. Unfortunately, though, there is an information alert that regularly pops up when "Straterra" is searched for on the Internet:

Strattera Suicide Risk in Children

Strattera may cause an increase in suicidal thoughts and actions in some children and teenagers, especially if your child has bipolar disorder or depression in addition to ADD/ADHD.

Call the doctor immediately if your child shows agitation, irritability, suicidal thinking or behaviors, and unusual changes in behavior.

Side Effects Associated with Non-Stimulant Medication

I would like to say that non-stimulants are much better than stimulants, as they are not classified as Schedule II narcotics the way stimulants are. But unfortunately, they too have a slew of side effects that include all of the following:

- dizziness
- fainting or feeling light-headed after getting up from a sitting or lying down position
- fatigue
- headache
- heartburn, gas, loss of appetite, nausea, or vomiting
- hot flashes
- irritability or mood swings

- painful menstruation
- runny nose
- skin rash or itching, prickling, or tingling sensations on the skin
- trouble sleeping
- weight loss
- agitation
- aggressive behaviour
- increased blood pressure
- palpitations (feeling your heart beat quickly or irregularly)
- problems with urination
- symptoms of depression (e.g., losing interest in your usual activities, feeling sad, or having thoughts of suicide)
- symptoms of liver damage (e.g., yellow skin or eyes, abdominal pain, loss of appetite, pale stools, or dark urine)
- hallucinations (e.g., hearing, seeing, or sensing things that are not there)
- symptoms of a serious allergic reaction (e.g., hives, swelling of the face and throat, or difficulty breathing)
- thoughts of suicide or of hurting yourself
- suicide

I'm not going to say anything further about ADHD medications, as I think you get the picture and this is not what this book is about. But before you administer that first pill, whether or not you're the one taking it, just review the previous lists of side effects and ask yourself if it's really worth the risk.

THE MULTI-PRONGED APPROACH TO TREATING ADHD

We all want the easy way out when it comes to ADHD—the shortcuts, the magic pill, whatever it takes. Unfortunately, there is no such thing. ADHD cannot be "fixed" or "cured" in one fell swoop. But it doesn't have to take up all of your time, energy, and attention either. Once you have the infrastructure of a routine down pat, it works extremely well. The six main components of a secure multi-pronged approach are shown below:

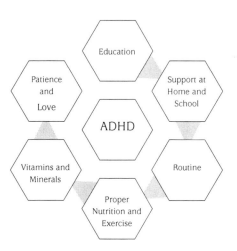

The Multi-Pronged Approach to ADHD

Some of these need explanation (nutrition and education), whereas others are no-brainers (patience and love). Once you have each of these established in your home and at your child's school, ADHD is entirely manageable without the terrifying side effects of medications gone wrong.

Let food be thy medicine and medicine be thy food.
—Hippocrates

DIET, NUTRITION, AND ADHD

Proper nutrition plays a complementary role in any person's life and especially in that of an individual struggling with ADHD. It is one of the more important segments of the multi-pronged approach to treating ADHD.

Simplified, when an individual's diet is balanced and healthy, his ADHD symptoms will be better controlled. It is extremely important as well to make dietary modifications for the entire family when changing the diet of the person with ADHD. No one wants to be singled out, especially a child or a teen, so support in the home is crucial.

Here are some easy tips to stick to. These are essential, so commit them to memory:

- Offer a variety of foods from as many food groups as possible at each meal or snack. The more colourful, the better.

- Encourage eating at regular intervals throughout the day. It helps keep concentration levels even and irritation at bay—this is also known as "grazing." Generally, children's behaviour often deteriorates in the late morning and late afternoon, or three to four hours after a meal, but incorporating grazing has many benefits, which include the following:
  - *better regulation of blood sugar levels*
  - *improved brain function*

- *controllable behaviour*
- *increased concentration levels*
- *ease in being able to incorporate the four fruit and five vegetable servings each day*
- *easier tactics for incorporating high-protein/low-carbohydrate mini meals*

Here are just a few ideas for mini meals and smart snacking tactics:

- *fruit*
- *veggies*
- *nuts (unsalted)*
- *popcorn (lightly salted)*
- *organic tortilla chips (unsalted or lightly salted) and organic salsa (salsa is extremely easy to make)*
- *pretzels*
- *smoothies*
- *trail mix*
- *organic peanut, almond, or cashew butter sandwich (or half sandwich), or any of these butters served with fruit and/or veggies*
- *aspartame-free yogurt (Greek yogurt is amazing)*
- *pickles*
- *natural granola bars (not chocolate-coated and not the "sweet and salty" variety)*
- *hummus or tzatziki with pita bread or veggies*
- *whole-grain cereal with or without milk*
- *popsicles made with natural fruit juice*
- *frozen grapes (these are amazing—just put some grapes in the freezer for a few hours and voilà!)*

- *cheese and crackers (whole-grain, low-salt crackers)*
- *edamame*

- Avoid any food items with added sugar at all costs. Foods that are especially high in processed sugars may spike blood sugar levels. This is called the "spike and crash syndrome." Additionally, sugar exacerbates ADHD immensely and makes symptoms worse, particularly hyperactivity.

- Refrain from serving any foods that have added food colouring and preservatives. Scientific studies have shown that food dyes can cause a significant increase in behavioural problems, such as hyperactivity, irritability, poor concentration, restlessness, and sleep disturbance. Additionally, one study showed a 70 percent improvement in symptoms when artificial food colouring was eliminated from the diets of both children and adults with ADHD. Remember this rule of thumb: If you can't pronounce it, don't buy it!

- Opt for a high-protein/low-carbohydrate diet that includes eggs, meat, nuts, and beans. This will improve concentration levels immensely and decrease sugar levels (carbohydrates convert to sugar, which can aid in spiking sugar levels).

- Try to opt for organic whenever possible. There are foods that should be bought organic and foods that should not. Here is a list of the most common items to simplify things for you:

Buy Organic	Don't Buy Organic
potatoes	onions
peanut butter	bananas
milk	pineapples
apples	avocados
meat	cabbage
nectarines	asparagus
spinach	mangoes
peaches	kiwis
pears	cantaloupe
strawberries	watermelons
bell peppers	sweet potatoes
eggs	mushrooms
grapes	honey
dairy products	grapefruit

If you're unsure if the produce you are buying is organic or not, the sticker or label attached to the fruit or vegetable will let you know. This is called a "PLU – Price Lookup" code and not only does it determine the price of the produce, but how it was grown as well:

- If there are only **four numbers** in the PLU code, this indicates that the item was grown **conventionally** with the use of pesticides.
- If there are **five numbers** in the PLU code, and the number starts with "**8**," this tells you that the item is a **genetically modified** fruit or vegetable.
- If there are **five numbers** in the PLU code, and the number starts with "**9**," this tells you that the item was grown **organically**.

Note: Organic foods tend to go bad much faster than inorganic foods, so be sure either to purchase small quantities of them or eat them quickly. Additionally, organic foods will also have more bacteria a week after

*purchase, as organic farmers are usually less efficient in getting their
products to the market.*

- Stay away from frozen meals and any foods that are "convenient." Many of these meal varieties contain food dyes and preservatives as previously mentioned above. However, you are usually safe with frozen fruits and vegetables. Purchasing organic fruits and vegetables is also not too much more expensive than buying regular frozen fruits and vegetables.

- This is the most important tip: Stay away from sports drinks (e.g., Gatorade and Powerade), soda pop, Slurpees, slushies, etc. All of these contain not only various dyes but also all sorts of preservatives and sugars. Allowing your child—or yourself, for that matter—to drink these would be a very unwise decision. Make your own "Slurpees" by mixing natural fruit juice and ice in a blender, and swap sports drinks for filtered water with added fresh lemon or lime, or even a splash of natural fruit juice.

- Ensure that, when giving a "reward," it is in a small amount, and be mindful of what exactly you are giving.

"Don't ask why healthy food is so expensive. Ask yourself why junk food is so cheap!"

ADHD AND BEST NUTRITION PRACTICES

To reiterate, proper food and nutrition are crucial, whether or not you have ADHD. When a child, teen, or adult is diagnosed with ADHD, these factors become even *more* important, because essentially, food fuels the human brain.

- Food supports or inhibits learning, functioning, and behaviour.
- Healthy fats and oils are extremely important, as they are brain-building for kids.
- Omega-3 fatty acids should be consumed *daily* to aid in focus, whether by food or through supplements.
- Hidden sources of added sugar (i.e., Pop-Tarts, sports drinks, sugary cereals, etc.) should be replaced with whole-food versions.
- Iron-rich foods and supplements aid in learning (low iron levels make kids moody, less focused, sleepy, and they promote poor cognition).
- Poor iron intake also makes kids more irritable and hyper.
- Meals should be prepared from scratch as often as possible. This way, you know exactly what is in each meal.
- Meal plans that incorporate many small meals rather than three large ones help control the "highs and lows" during the course of the day.

- High-protein/low-carbohydrate diets are highly recommended for children, teens, and adults with ADHD.
  Protein-rich foods are used by the brain to make essential
  neurotransmitters.

  - *The body converts processed carbohydrates into glucose
    (sugar) so quickly that the effect is virtually the same as
    eating sugar straight from a spoon.*

  - *Combining protein with complex carbohydrates that are
    high in fibre and low in sugar will help your child manage
    his ADHD symptoms better during the day. Here is an
    example: organic peanut butter on a piece of whole-grain
    bread. The sugars from these carbohydrates are digested
    more slowly because protein, fibre, and fat eaten together
    result in a more gradual and sustained blood sugar release,
    rather than in sugar "spikes."*

MENU PLANNING 101

When people contemplate menu planning, they essentially think, "Ugh . . . more work!" But this isn't the case at all. Menu planning can be easy, fun, and quite simple. It's also a way of involving the entire family in the process so that every meal is a smashing success.

Try to think of menu planning more like this:

- It will ensure that convenience foods do not become so convenient.

- It will save money by reducing impulse spending and trips to the supermarket. Leftovers cut food waste, and buying in bulk makes it easy to stockpile freezer meals at reduced prices.

- It will save time. There will be no need to make a dash to the neighbours' for a missing ingredient, and no frantic searches through the freezer for something to thaw for dinner.

- It will improve nutrition. Without having to run to the supermarket, there will be time to prepare side dishes and salads to complement the main dish, which will increase the family's consumption of fruits and vegetables. Knowing what to serve each day and already having the ingredients on hand will cut back on the drive-through habit as well.

Other important things to note about menu planning include these tips:

- Post the menu plan on the refrigerator door once you have put it together. Refer to it during the coming week as you prepare meals.

- Build a personal shopping list but have an open mind when shopping. Menu plans aren't written in stone, so stay flexible to avoid stress.

- Create a routine around your menu planning. Routine is important for your children, so make it important for you as well.

- Make menu planning a habit—a menu plan won't help you if you don't make one.

- Recycle menu plans. Once you have already done four or five weeks, start from week one again.

- Menu plan by season. Fruits and vegetables are much easier to buy when the ingredients are actually in season. Additionally, seasonal fruits and vegetables are more cost-effective.

- Don't get too stressed out; menu planning should be fun! Ask the family for ideas of what they would like to see on the menu.

- Build flexibility into your menu plan on the off chance that you forget to purchase something or time just won't allow you to make what you had originally planned.

- Ensure each meal has every food group.

- Ensure that each dish is easy to prepare. Save more difficult dishes, such as lasagna, for a day when you are not working and you actually have time to make it properly.

- Write your shopping list once you've planned your meals. This will simplify your shopping immensely.

- Go through cookbooks and be sure to utilize the Internet for interesting ideas.
- Let each person pick a meal, and most importantly, let each person actually make a meal. If a family member is too young, then have that person help.

Please refer to the Appendix for a one-week sample meal plan.

NUTRITION LABELLING

I will not go into nutrition labelling in full, as there are only basics that you need to know.

Nutrition labelling became mandatory in Canada and in the United States for all prepackaged foods on December 12, 2007, and is required by law. Food labels were developed as a general guide to help people choose foods wisely and understand what is actually in a product itself. Reading nutrition labels can assist you in deciding which products are best for you.

Why Nutrition Labelling Is Important to You

The information on a nutrition label includes the following:
- a Nutrition Facts table that lists calories, thirteen core nutrients, and % Daily Value (%DV) of nutrients
- the list of ingredients
- some optional nutrition claims

All of the information in the Nutrition Facts table is based on a specific amount of food found at the top of the table.

Nutrition Facts

Serving Size 2/3 cup (51g)
Servings Per Container About 9

Amount Per Serving	Cereal	Cereal with 1/2 cup Skim Milk
Calories	240	280
Calories from Fat	70	70
	% Daily Value**	
Total Fat 8g*	12%	12%
Saturated Fat 2.5g	13%	13%
Trans Fat 0g		
Cholesterol 0mg	0%	0%
Sodium 50mg	2%	5%
Total Carbohydrate 37g	12%	14%
Dietary Fiber 3g	12%	12%
Sugars 13g		
Protein 4g	8%	16%
Vitamin A	0%	4%
Vitamin C	0%	0%
Calcium	2%	15%
Iron	6%	6%

But have you ever wondered what the difference between "reduced fat" and "low fat" is, or what "calorie free" on a label really means? Health Canada and the Food and Drug Administration have strict guidelines as to how these food label terms can be used.

Here are some of the most common claims seen on food packages and what these terms mean:

- **Low Calorie:** has 40 calories or less per serving
- **Low Cholesterol:** has 20 milligrams or less and also 2 grams or less of saturated fat per serving
- **Reduced:** has at least 25 percent less of the specified nutrient or calories than the usual product
- **Good Source Of:** provides at least 10 to 19 percent of the Daily Value of a particular vitamin or nutrient per serving
- **Calorie Free:** has 5 calories or less per serving
- **Fat Free/Sugar Free:** has ½ gram or less of fat or sugar per serving
- **Low Sodium:** has 140 milligrams or less of sodium per serving
- **High In:** provides 20 percent or more of the Daily Value of a specified nutrient per serving
- **High Fibre:** has 5 grams or more of fibre per serving

For some people, interpreting nutrition labels can seem tricky. But it doesn't have to be. Below is an easy way to figure out whether or not something would be a healthy snack.

Snack items that boast having only "100 calories" are a big deal right now, but do you know what those calories are really made up of? Let's have a look at a popular cheddar popcorn treat—that delicious white cheddar popcorn that is so light it almost floats out of the bag when opened. It can't be that bad for you, can it?

But take this into consideration:

1 gram of fat = 9 calories
1 gram of protein = 4 calories
1 gram of carbohydrates = 4 calories

So according to their food label,
$$\text{total fat} = 6 \text{ grams}$$
$$\text{total carbohydrates} = 9 \text{ grams}$$
$$\text{total protein} = 2 \text{ grams}$$

And therefore,
$$\text{total calories from fat} = 54 \text{ calories}$$
(*half* the calories come from fat!)
$$\text{total calories from carbs} = 36 \text{ calories}$$
$$\text{total calories from protein} = 8 \text{ calories}$$

So the actual calorie count is 108 calories, not 100. Plus, half the calories come from fat, and in this particular case, not a good fat either. Definitely not a wise choice when snacking.

Not all commercial snack food is like this, but this is the simplest way to break down your three prime nutrients when you're in a hurry.

HOW TO GROCERY SHOP AND BE SUPERMARKET SAVVY

People think that shopping is easy, but in essence, it isn't. It's easy, yes, to buy all the wrong items but hard to find what's nutritious. Here are some key points to keep in mind when grocery shopping:

- Shop the perimeter of the grocery store, where fresh foods such as fruits, vegetables, dairy, meat, and fish are usually located. Avoid the centre aisles, where junk foods lurk.

- Choose "real" foods such as 100 percent fruit juice or 100 percent whole-grain items with as few processed ingredients and additives as possible. If you want more salt or sugar, add it yourself.

- Steer clear of foods with cartoons on the labels that are targeted to children. If you don't want your kids eating junk foods, *don't have these items in the house.*

- Avoid foods that contain more than five ingredients, artificial ingredients, or ingredients you can't pronounce.

- **Produce:** Spend the most time in the produce section. Choose a rainbow of colourful fruits and vegetables. The colours reflect the different vitamin, mineral, and phytonutrient contents of each fruit or vegetable.

- **Breads, Cereals, and Pastas:** Choose whole-grain

products over any other foods, especially processed foods. For example, regular oatmeal is preferable to instant oatmeal due to the high sugar content in the latter.

- *Breads, pastas, rice, and grains offer more opportunities to work whole-grains into your diet. Choose whole-wheat breads and pastas, brown rice, grain mixes, quinoa, bulgur, and barley. To help your family get used to whole-grains, you can start out with whole-wheat blends and slowly transition to 100 percent whole-wheat pastas and breads.*

- **Meat, Fish, and Poultry:** Canada's Food Guide recommends two servings of fish per week. Salmon is an excellent source of Omega-3 fatty acids. Be sure to choose lean cuts of meat (such as round, top sirloin, and tenderloin), opt for skinless poultry, and watch your portion sizes.

- **Dairy:** Dairy foods are an excellent source of bone-building calcium and vitamin D. There are plenty of low-fat and nonfat options to help you get three servings a day, including drinkable and single-serve tube yogurts, and pre-portioned cheeses. If you enjoy higher-fat cheeses, no problem—just keep your portions small.

- **Frozen Foods:** Frozen fruits and vegetables (without sauce) are a convenient way to help fill in the produce gap, especially in winter. But double-check the ingredients—if you don't know what it is, don't buy it!

- **Canned and Dried Foods:** Keep a variety of canned vegetables, fruits, and beans on hand to toss into soups, salads, pastas, or rice dishes. Whenever possible, choose vegetables without added salt as well as fruit packed in juice. Tuna packed in water, low-fat soups, nut butters, olive and canola oils, and assorted vinegars should be in every healthy pantry.

CONVENIENCE VS. HOMEMADE

This is a no-brainer: Homemade dishes (meaning dishes made from scratch) are better for you than convenience items for many reasons. There are several pros and cons for each, and sometimes, it is just easier to have one over the other and vice versa. With that being said, choose wisely. Choose your meals wisely, your recipes wisely, and your time wisely—when shopping *and* when cooking. These will be your three biggest components when deciding between convenience and homemade foods.

Pros and Cons of Convenience Foods

PROS	CONS
There is usually less time required for food preparation.	They may be higher in fat, making their energy (calorie) content high.
There are usually fewer dishes and utensils being used.	They are often higher in sodium because sodium is a cheap flavour.
The meals have consistent flavour, so there are no changes from time to time.	The cook cannot control the ingredients of the product, which makes it much harder to control the sugar, fat, and salt content.
There is little skill required to heat or prepare the meal.	They allow for little recipe modification, as the meal is already prepared.
	They are most often processed or contain processed ingredients.
	The ingredients can generally be unknown, frozen, unpronounceable, etc.

Pros and Cons of Homemade Foods

PROS	CONS
They are less expensive than mixes.	There is usually more time involved in preparing and cooking the meal.
There is more creativity and freedom with the ingredients included in the dish.	There are more dishes and utensils used, which makes cleanup a lengthy process.
The cook can improve quality and flavour with ingredient choices.	
The cook has the option to reduce or eliminate fat and salt in recipes.	
The cook knows *exactly* all the ingredients used to make the food.	
The ingredients are generally fresh.	
The cook takes more pride in each meal.	
There is more fun involved when preparing meals, especially when other family members, such as children, are included in the process.	

So regardless of your choice, please check your nutrition labels carefully and remember what Julia Child once said: "You don't have to cook fancy or complicated masterpieces—just good food from fresh ingredients."

ADHD AND ENVIRONMENTAL TOXINS, ADDITIVES, AND FOOD DYES

There has been study after study on the link between environmental toxins, additives in foods, food dyes, and ADHD. Notably, the most prevalent study has shown that children exposed to certain toxins are at increased risk of behavioural problems. The exposure can come in various forms, some of which you would least expect!

Below is a list of some interesting information on this correlation:

- Exposure to lead, found mainly in paint and pipes in older buildings, has been linked to disruptive (and even violent) behaviour and to short attention spans in children.

- Pregnant women who are exposed to environmental toxins such as tobacco, alcohol, and illicit drugs may reduce the activity of vital nerve cells (neurons) in the brain. These neurons produce neurotransmitters in the baby's brain that will then increase the baby's risk of being born with ADHD.

- In a 2007 study by Michigan State University, scientists found that children who had ADHD had higher levels of lead in their blood. Elevated lead levels may make it harder for the brain to develop, thus making it difficult for children to regulate their self-control.

- In the same study by Michigan State University, scientists found that exposure to pesticides through food can cause children to have substantially higher levels of neurotoxic organophosphate pesticides, which will then make them twice as likely to be diagnosed with ADHD.

- There has been additional research that has shown the importance of women eating organic foods, particularly produce, at least six months before conception and throughout pregnancy.

- Substances added to food, such as artificial colouring or food preservatives, may contribute to hyperactive behaviour.

- Studies in Canada, the USA, and the UK have found a definite link between food additives and behaviour problems in children, such as temper tantrums and poor concentration. Because several studies have looked at a combination of food additives and their possible effects on hyperactivity and ADHD, it isn't clear which additives specifically might affect behaviour.

- Some food additives, though, that have been shown to increase hyperactive behaviour include the following:

  - **Sodium Benzoate** *(food preservative): commonly used in fruit pies, jams, beverages, salads, relishes, and sauerkraut*

  - **Blue No. 1** *(Brilliant Blue): commonly used in some Yoplait products, some Jell-O dessert products, Fruity Cheerios, Froot Loops, some Pop-Tarts products, some Oscar Mayer Lunchables, Duncan Hines Whipped Chocolate Frosting, Skittles candy, Jolly Rancher Screaming Sours Soft & Chewy Candy, Eclipse gum, and Fanta grape soda*

  - **Blue No. 2** *(Indigotine): commonly used in Froot Loops, Pop-Tarts products, Duncan Hines Moist Deluxe Straw-*

berry Supreme Premium Cake Mix, Betty Crocker Rich & Creamy Cherry Frosting, M&M's milk chocolate candy, M&M's milk chocolate peanut candy, and Wonka Nerds grape and strawberry flavoured candy

- **Green No. 3**: *rarely used, but can still be found in some candy, beverages, ice creams, and puddings*
- **Orange B**: *rarely used, but can still be found in some sausage casings*
- **Red No. 3** *(Carmoisine): found in some candy, cake icing, and chewing gum*
- **Red No. 40** *(Allura Red): by far the most popular and commonly used in some Yoplait products, some Jello-O dessert products, Quaker Instant Oatmeal, Froot Loops, Trix, some Pop-Tarts products, Oscar Mayer Lunchables, Hostess Twinkies, some Pillsbury rolls and frostings, some Betty Crocker and Duncan Hines frostings, and more*
- **Yellow No. 5** *(Tartrazine): commonly used in Nabisco Cheese Nips Four Cheese crackers, Hunt's Snack Pack Pudding products, Lucky Charms, Eggo waffle and other waffle products, some Pop-Tarts products, various Kraft macaroni-and-cheese products, Betty Crocker products, Hamburger Helper products, and more (This food dye has been tested alone and has a direct link to hyperactivity.)*
- **Yellow No. 6** *(Sunset Yellow): commonly used in Betty Crocker Fruit Roll-Ups, some Jell-O dessert products and instant puddings, Fruity Cheerios, Trix, some Eggo waffle products, some Kraft macaroni-and-cheese products, Betty Crocker frostings, some M&M's and Skittles candy, Sunkist orange soda, and Fanta orange soda*

Sadly, many food colourings and food additives don't require labelling other than Yellow No. 5. Food dyes are currently banned in the UK, and more and more companies are looking to natural products, such as plants, to add colour. The USA has banned some of the food dyes but still uses a fair number of them. The same is true for Canada.

SUPPLEMENTS 101

Over the past few decades, alternative and complementary medicine has grown in popularity all over the world. Although many people argue this fact, especially doctors and psychiatrists, supplements are a necessary component in supporting brain chemistry. There are various remedies used in the place of standard medical approaches that are considered safe, relatively affordable, and easily accessible. Please remember, before administering any supplement to your child or to yourself, it is incredibly important to check with a pediatrician or doctor. This is because some natural or alternative remedies can be unsafe.

In order for a supplement to have full effect, it must be administered, like a medicine, generally at the same time each day. Additionally, in order to notice any effects, be sure to give the supplement at least two weeks to really kick in.

Below is a list of supplements that are effective for children, teenagers, and adults and a breakdown of what each one's primary goal is. As for getting an adequate RDI (Recommended Daily Intake), the values listed below are for children and adolescents, so if you are an adult, again, check with your doctor or naturopath as to the best dosage for you. Additionally, I have included the best sources of these vitamins and supplements for those who absolutely despise or generally have a hard time taking pills of any sort.

And finally, one last tip: The best time to take any vitamin or supplement is in the morning. This is because the body is deprived of nutrients and requires energy to function during the day. Generally, vitamins should be taken within thirty minutes after eating a healthy breakfast containing protein, calcium, and fruit. Consuming vitamins while eating food helps ensure that they are processed by the body, as they will be broken down and digested along with the food. Taking your vitamins in the morning also ensures that their nutrients are used effectively throughout the day. If, perchance, you forget to take your vitamins in the morning, don't sweat it—just take them at lunchtime or forego them that day altogether and make sure your diet contains the vitamins vital to good health.

SUPPLEMENTS

Thiamine
- helps improve behaviour
- dosing starts at 25–50 milligrams per day
- best sources include tuna, beans, fortified breakfast cereals, Brussels sprouts, sunflower seeds, pork chops, pistachios, macadamia nuts, pecans, brown rice, asparagus, kale, potatoes, eggs, liver (beef, pork, chicken), and marmite (yeast extract)

Niacin (Vitamin B3)
- helps in alleviating symptoms of hyperactivity and weakening school performance; assists in maintaining social relationships
- dosing starts at 10 milligrams per day
- best sources include wheat bran, pork chops, chicken, tuna, salmon, mackerel, trout, herring, sardines, beef, peanuts, fortified breakfast cereals, marmite (yeast extract), liver, paprika, sun-dried tomatoes, mushrooms, potatoes, and cottage cheese

Pyridoxine (Vitamin B6)
- highly effective at treating hyperactivity
- dosing starts at 25 milligrams per day
- best sources include wheat bran, pistachios, raw garlic,

liver, tuna, salmon, mackerel, cod, halibut, trout, sunflower
seeds, sesame seeds, pork, molasses, hazelnuts, potatoes,
sweet potatoes, carrots, avocados, and soy beverages

Magnesium

- aids in alleviating excessive fidgeting, anxiety, and restlessness
- dosing starts at 100 milligrams per day
- best sources include spinach, potatoes, okra, fortified
  breakfast cereals, soy beverages, tofu, sunflower seeds,
  hummus, almonds, cashews, pine nuts, flaxseeds, peanuts,
  salmon, halibut, mackerel, pollack, and crab

Calcium

- aids in alleviating hyperactivity
- dosing starts at 1,000 milligrams per day
- best sources include spinach, kale, turnip greens, milk
  products, cheese, yogurt, salmon, mackerel, sardines, anchovies, tofu, almonds, and molasses

Zinc

- aids in reducing hyperactivity, impulsivity, and irritability
- dosing starts at 10 milligrams per day
- best sources include wheat germ, cereal, milk, cheese,
  yogurt, liver, beef, veal, lamb, turkey, pork, chicken, baked
  beans, pine nuts, peanuts, cashews, almonds, lentils, eggs,
  oysters, scallops, lobster, clams, mussels, anchovies, and
  shrimp

Iron

- aids in reducing irritability and improving attentiveness
  and memory
- dosing starts at 25 milligrams per day

- best sources include clams, oysters, liver, squash, pumpkin seeds, cashews, hazelnuts, peanuts, almonds, beef, lamb, beans, whole-grains, spinach, Swiss chard, tofu, and dark chocolate

Omega-3

- aids in improving focus, mood, and memory; helps alleviate temper tantrums and sleep problems
- dosing starts at 700–1,500 milligrams per day, depending on the weight of the child
- best sources include wheat germ, squash, radish, edamame, fortified milk and yogurt, eggs, anchovies, caviar, clams, cod, mackerel, lobster, halibut, mussels, oysters, salmon, sardines, trout, tuna, snapper, beans, pecans, flaxseed, walnuts, and almonds

The key here is to incorporate all the food groups when eating and make your plate of food as colourful as possible. This will introduce an incredible amount of vitamins and supplements as well as various textures and flavours into your diet.

Additionally, pill form or liquid form is always suggested over gummy form. This is because the gummy varieties of vitamins contain food colouring, other additives, and sugar. The vitamin content in these is much lower than that of a pill or liquid, where it is much more concentrated.

Physical fitness is not only one of the most important keys to a healthy body, it is the basis of dynamic and creative intellectual activity.
—John F. Kennedy

ADHD AND EXERCISE

I don't have to tell you that exercise is important for several reasons, and, as an adult, you either love it or hate it. But when it comes to children, we all have to set examples of ourselves and model exercise in a positive light. This includes making it fun, mixing it up, showing incredible support, and educating wherever possible.

Below are some of the most important reasons exercise must be incorporated into everyone's life, *every single day*—especially in the life of someone who struggles with ADHD.

- Hormone-like compounds in our system are released when we exercise. These are called endorphins. These endorphins regulate moods such as pleasure and pain. Other compounds, or chemicals, that are released during exercise are in the brain. They include dopamine, norepinephrine, and serotonin. The levels of these compounds are elevated during exercise and, when raised, aid in supporting focus, attention, and alertness, and improve poor social skills.

- To release restless energy, which can be negative and bothersome for teachers, parents, coaches, and tutors, kids with ADHD need to get plenty of exercise. Sometimes, physical activity done in as little as twenty-minute spurts can do the trick.

- Studies have shown that exercise can have many of the same effects on children with ADHD as stimulant drugs.

- Kids with ADHD who exercise also perform better on tests of attention and have less impulsivity.

- Exercise also increases blood flow to the brain, which, in turn, aids with the following:

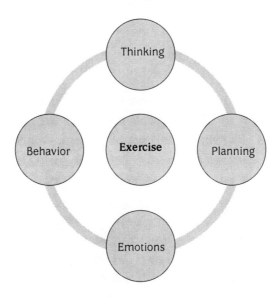

The effect of exercise on the human body

- Additionally, kids who exercise get in trouble less often for disruptive behaviours such as talking out of turn, name calling, hitting, moving inappropriately, and refusing to participate in activities.

Individual sports, such as tennis or karate, and team sports, such as soccer, football, or baseball, offer great ways for your child to exercise. Either way, encourage both with your child. If he finds a sport that he particularly loves, roll with it! This means that he has found something that he truly loves and enjoys, so encourage him as much as possible.

ADHD AND SLEEP

Sleep disturbances are a common problem for ADHDer's as they not only keep them from falling asleep, but also staying asleep throughout the night. This could be due to several factors which include:
- the ability to turn off their brain at the end of the day
- their restlessness which they have a hard time containing
- their hyperactivity level which they haven't had a chance to calm down prior to going to bed
- any comorbid condition they may have in addition to their ADHD (such as anxiety or depression)
- stimulant medication that they could be taking

There are several ways to aid in problematic sleep disturbances but consulting with their doctor should be first and foremost. In my experience, routine works immensely. Factors that work extremely well and should be part of their routine include:
- setting the same time to go to bed each night
- taking away any electronics one hour prior to bedtime and keeping TV's, computers and cell phones out of the bedroom
- having a hot bath or shower
- eliminating eating late in the evening
- making their bedroom conducive to sleep – dark, cool and quiet

- avoiding sleeping in on the weekends
- eliminating naps during the day
- sticking to a nutritious diet

If none of these suggestions work, a melatonin supplement can work well (3 mg tablet) but **please consult your child's doctor prior to administering it** as individuals react differently to such supplements. It should also be noted that melatonin should be a last resort and not be taken long term or on a daily basis. (Melatonin is a hormone found in plants and animals and is important in helping regulate the internal body clock's cycle of sleep and wakefulness.) Sleeping pills (for example, benzodiazepines), are sometimes prescribed for adults with sleeping problems, but their **effects in children haven't been studied enough.** And please note that it is never safe to give your child medication prescribed for someone else.

For people with ADHD, getting a good night's sleep is important as poor sleep (too little sleep or symptoms of sleep disorders) may profoundly impact ADHD symptoms. Treating sleep problems may also help decrease, or sometimes eliminate, attention and hyperactivity issues for some children.

ADHD COACHING

ADHD coaching is a relatively new field but is becoming increasingly popular throughout North America. Generally, an ADHD coach will work with individuals of all ages to help them reach their full potential in all aspects of their lives. These professionals have a distinct understanding of how ADHD affects their clients and of the challenges those with ADHD and their families are faced with daily.

ADHD coaches also help keep their clients accountable and will provide support in many facets, such as the following:

- setting goals
- increasing confidence
- building motivation
- focusing
- prioritizing
- organizing
- scheduling
- identifying passions and talents
- utilizing ADHD characteristics (e.g., hyper-focusing, creative thinking, etc.)
- figuring out what to do when "stuck" (e.g., dealing with distraction, time management issues, perfectionism, and procrastination)

ADHD coaching isn't for everyone, and as an ADHDer, you either love it or you hate it. Many people don't like it, as they're not ready for coaching or they don't actually want a coach (which I translate to "I don't want help" because they're not willing to do the work). But, in fact, if you have the right coach, this system works extremely well.

Consider these tips:

- For ADHD children and teens, an ADHD coach is almost like a "big buddy," so finding the right fit is important.

- ADHD coaches help the client clarify what is problematic, and they break down problems into definable goals with steps the client can take.

- An ADHD coach does not and should not deal with psychological and emotional issues (such as drug addiction or depression) but will provide sensible and achievable strategies that will help in day-to-day life. ADHD coaching is not therapy and, therefore, should not be treated as such.

- ADHD coaches also keep clients accountable and provide support. This is an extremely important factor in ADHD coaching, as accountability is crucial for anyone who struggles with ADHD.

If you're still unsure whether or not having an ADHD coach is right for you, take into account these clues that will indicate if you or your child will benefit from working with a coach:

- You acknowledge that your child is capable of so much more, and you feel that with a little help, he will be "on par" with his friends or classmates.

- You see that your child has aspirations and goals, but he is not motivated to try to aspire toward them or does not even know where to start.

- Keeping your child organized is a full-time job and executive functioning is a continuous struggle.

- "Overwhelming" seems to be a term that is constantly expressed either verbally or physically.

- Procrastination is a constant struggle with most matters, such as chores, schoolwork, etc.

- Your child appears scattered quite often and with a real need for direction.

- Various aspects of your child's life tend to get neglected, such as personal hygiene, homework, friends, exercise, etc.

- Life is unbalanced and the negative habits overpower the positive habits.

- "Follow-through" is another constant battle. Many tasks do get started but are then rarely finished.

- Frustration is constant, turning into anxiety and then, possibly, other comorbid conditions.

A good ADHD coach can definitely help in many, many ways. Here is what you should look for when seeking the right coach:

- Search on reputable sites that provide a national directory of coaches throughout North America. Once you have found someone in your area, check out her website to ensure her professionalism, accreditation, etc.

- Check out the coach's background. Pay careful attention to her education, the number of years she has been coaching, and her level of training.

- Consider testimonials. These are important and some coaches even allow for you to contact a reference.

- Be sure to interview the coach and address any questions or concerns you may have. Make sure you understand what you need help with and how an ADHD coach can assist.

- Don't feel pressured to make a decision on the spot. If

you're still undecided, take time to think things through. Remember that this is an investment in your child or you, so you want to be comfortable paying for services that you truly believe in.

- Have reasonable expectations when interviewing the ADHD coach. The ADHD coach is just that—a coach. She is not a tutor, a therapist, a psychiatrist, or a counsellor. She is there to serve as a guide to help you or your child understand more about ADHD while discovering new skills, habits, and strategies.

- Lastly, trust your gut! If it seems that something just doesn't feel right, then stick to it. You know your child or yourself best as well as what will work and not work.

ADHD coaching is usually done one-on-one by phone, Skype, and/or e-mail. A time commitment is essential, as the average amount of time it takes to see a change is approximately three months. In order to establish a sound coaching relationship and achieve long-term success, a minimum commitment of six months is suggested.

ADD is like going through life, carrying a one-man-band contraption with a broken strap.
—Julia Smith-Ruetz

ADHD AND EXECUTIVE FUNCTION

The term "executive function" has a certain ring to it—it almost sounds like something that only businesspeople have problems with, but this is furthest from the truth. In a nutshell, executive function refers to a set of mental skills that work together in the frontal lobe of the brain and help a person achieve goals. These brain functions activate, organize, integrate, and manage other functions.

The goals of executive function include the following:

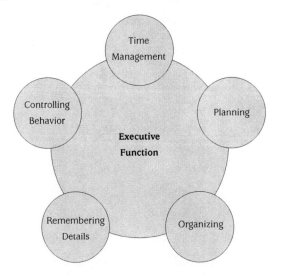

Goals of Executive Function

When executive function breaks down, behaviour becomes poorly managed and will affect someone's ability to fulfill these tasks and responsibilities:

- working
- attending school
- keeping social relationships
- behaving independently

Executive function problems can run in the family and will become most evident during a child's elementary school years. This is the time when they interfere with the child's ability to start and complete schoolwork on time, when items get lost on a regular basis, and when the concept of time eludes the child.

There are warning signs to look out for that show that a child may be having difficulty with executive function. These include indicators that the child is experiencing trouble in accomplishing the types of actions listed below:

- planning projects
- telling stories (either verbally or in writing)
- memorizing information
- estimating how much time an activity or project will take to complete
- commencing or starting tasks or activities
- retaining information during the process of doing something with that information (an example would be remembering a phone number while dialing that number)
- chronically "forgetting" to bring homework home or identifying that there is actually homework

There is no single test to identify if there is a problem with executive function, but teachers, speech-language pathologists, counsellors, and therapists rely on different tests to measure specific skills. Usually, careful observation and trial teaching are more valuable ways of identifying and improving weak executive function.

Coping with Poor Executive Function Skills

If you suspect that there are problems with the executive function of your child, it's best to nip them in the bud at an early age. Here are some general things to try:

- Use specific tools, such as watches with alarms, agendas, and organizers.
- Use visual schedules and review them consistently throughout the day.
- Take baby steps when approaching work. Using visual aids works best and is very reliable.
- Ask that the directions be repeated so that the instruction is instilled.
- Structure and plan shifts for various activities (for example, spend twenty minutes on one project, and when the timer goes off, move on to the next project).

Below are specific strategies for handling the various aspects of executive function.

To Improve Space Management and to Keep Things from Getting Lost

- Diminish clutter.
- Have separate work areas for different activities. Ensure that each work area has its own set of supplies.
- Organize the work space. Use various mini bins and labels to ensure that there is a place for everything.
- Ensure that the work space is cleaned weekly (schedule a specific time each week to do this).

To Improve Time Management

- Create checklists and to-do lists continuously. Also, make an estimate of how long each task will take.

- Do each task and assignment in small time frames, or "chunks." Assign each chunk a specific amount of time, and set a goal for completing it.

- Make sure that due dates are clear for each assignment or activity.

- Use visual calendars to keep track of the due dates of assignments, appointments, activities, and chores. Ensure that the calendar is large enough that it won't go unnoticed, and that it is placed somewhere it can always be seen (such as the kitchen). Visuals are extremely helpful for those who lack adequate executive function skills.

To Improve Work Habits

- Make a checklist when working on assignments. For example, a student's checklist could include such items: "get pen and pencil ready," "put name on paper," "put due date on paper," "read directions," etc. Again, using visuals can be very effective.

- Meet with the teacher on a regular basis to review work and troubleshoot problems. If this is done routinely, there will be little room for error.

- Hire an ADHD coach to establish accountability and keep things on track. This coach won't be needed forever, but just until some good habits are developed. Enlisting the assistance of an ADHD coach is a definite benefit and exceptional investment.

ADHD AND SCHOOL STRATEGIES

For many reasons, school can be *the* most frustrating experience for anyone with ADHD. Sitting still, paying attention, listening quietly, following instructions, and concentrating are definitely not easy, but by working with your child's teachers and school, you can come up with some great solutions to combat the challenges that ADHD causes and plant a firm track for success. There are many strategies that are simple but go a long way in helping your child have a positive and productive school experience.

All children need structure, but children with ADHD need it that much more. Trying to keep such a child organized is the hardest job in the world and a constant source of frustration. There is hope, though, as long as three specific criteria are met: finding the right tools for meeting the specific needs and goals of the child, long-term family commitment in using the required systems, and long-term school commitment in using the required systems.

Here are some key ways to help your ADHD child with school:

- Talk to your child's teacher or write his teacher a letter about your child's personality and learning style (please see the Appendix for a sample letter).
- Offer the teacher materials to help her learn more about ADHD.

- Work out a system for receiving regular reports.
- Help your ADHD child get organized—and stay organized (this is ongoing).
- Focus on the physical environment.
- Develop tools to ease tough transitions.
- Limit options—too many choices can be overwhelming both at home and at school.
- Avoid ADHD stigmas.
- Plan ahead.
- Make meetings happen.
- Create goals together (both with your child and with the teacher).
- Praise and encourage.
- Listen carefully.
- Help talent flourish.
- Share information.
- Ask the hard questions to get a complete picture.

Keeping an open line of communication with the teacher is vital and is best met depending on the situation at hand.

When the Key Issue Is Distractibility

- Make a request to the teacher to seat your child away from doors and windows. Put pets in another room or a corner while the student is working.
- Ask the teacher to alternate seated activities with those that allow your child to move his body around the room. Whenever possible, it's important to incorporate physical movement into lessons.
- Have the teacher write important information down where the child can easily read and reference it. Have the

teacher remind your child where this information can be found.

- Ask the teacher to divide big assignments into smaller ones and to allow your child frequent breaks.

When the Key Issue Is Impulsivity

- Ensure that a written behaviour plan is near your child.
- Ask the teacher to issue consequences immediately following misbehaviour. Ensure that the teacher is specific in her explanation, making sure your child knows how he misbehaved.
- Request that the teacher recognize good behaviour out loud. She should be specific in her praise, making sure your child knows what he did right.
- Have the teacher write the schedule for the day on a piece of paper and cross off each item as it is completed. Children with impulse problems may gain a sense of control and feel calmer when they know what to expect.

When the Key Issues Are Fidgeting and Hyperactivity

- Have the teacher ask your child to run an errand or do a task for her, even if it just means walking across the room to sharpen pencils or put dishes away.
- Ask the teacher to encourage your child to play a sport— or to at least run around before and after school.
- Provide the teacher with a stress ball, small toy, or other object for your child to squeeze or play with discreetly at his seat.
- Make sure your child *never* misses recess or PE.

It's important to work *with* the teacher and not against her. As the saying goes, you get more bees with honey!

Dealing with the Never-Ending Homework Issue

No one really likes homework, especially children and adolescents. Let me rephrase that—especially children and adolescents *with ADHD!*

Having ADHD can be tough, most notably when it comes to executive function (please refer to "ADHD and Executive Function"), so tackling homework on a daily basis is tiresome. Sometimes even just getting the assignment written down or getting the appropriate books in the knapsack to take home can be overwhelming. Papers get lost, assignments and homework don't get written down, or when they do, are usually incorrect, so trying to recall what the teacher said can prove frustrating.

Homework involves many steps. One missed step can create many problems. For the student, it can become so overwhelming that it is easier just not to do the homework. Homework can be frustrating for parents, children, tutors, and the teacher.

High school years can be an especially hard time for many reasons:

- Students have many teachers with various teaching styles.
- Students are under less supervision than they were in elementary school.
- The expectations held of the student are much higher, and their responsibilities are far greater.
- The student's self-esteem is more fragile, and feelings of self-consciousness rise.

But there are strategies to help the student with school and many ways that parents can assist as well.

Advocacy

This is, by far, one of the most important aspects in helping your child with school. You will need to advocate for your child regularly by meeting with the teacher or communicating with the teacher either by phone or by e-mail to discuss classroom or homework concerns.

It is important for your child's teacher to know exactly *how* to deal with your child, or with any child who has ADHD. Ensure that you find out what her knowledge base is regarding ADHD, and if the teacher knows very little, educate her. The more she knows, the easier it will be for all parties: the teacher, your child, and you.

Be sure also to advise the teacher of any strategies that you use with your child that genuinely work. For example, if you find that your child studies best listening to music, ask the teacher to allow your child to do quizzes and tests while listening to music. Although ADHD is not yet in the same category as a learning disability, consider asking if your child can be given extended time to complete assignments or exams. Most teachers should be on board with this idea, but if not, speak to the principal to put this strategy into place.

Textbooks

Forgetting textbooks for homework is inevitably going to happen, so ensure that you speak with your child's school about getting a second set of textbooks to keep at home during the school year. Children with ADHD struggle immensely when it comes to the end of the school day, and having a backup set at home can be a lifesaver on those more disorganized days.

Tools and Support

Routine is one of the most important aspects to keeping an ADHDer organized, so having the proper tools and support is vital. Some simple tools that go a long way are these:

- a notebook/agenda where homework assignments can be written down
- a dry-erase board or chalkboard for the bedroom
- an iPod (if your child works well while listening to music)
- fidgets (such as a stress ball) to use either at home or in the classroom

Ask the teacher as well regarding what strategies she has found to work in the classroom, and ask that you are informed of any upcoming quizzes, tests, assignments, or projects.

Backpack Organization

The backpack is the lifeline of any student, so help your child organize his backpack. Make "backpack organization" a part of homework time to help teach your child how to clean out old and unnecessary items in the backpack and keep any items that are needed daily (such as a water bottle or a house key). Having an organized backpack will help your child get his materials more efficiently and not get distracted by unnecessary items that are taking up space. This task may seem simple and small, but for a child with ADHD, it is huge. So having that extra support is imperative.

Colour Coding

Colour coding is extremely helpful, as most children are visual. For example, when purchasing notebooks or binders for school, designate red for language arts, blue for math, green for science, etc. Even colour code the pens. Additionally, buy a separate folder to store homework papers that match each notebook or binder. This folder will provide your child with a consistent place to store his homework papers and hopefully keep them from getting lost.

Structure Homework Time

One extremely good habit is to have your child do his homework soon after he comes home from school or from his after-school activities. Give him a snack first to nourish his brain and re-energize him, and then, it's homework time. Studies have shown that kids benefit greatly from as little as twenty minutes of exercise or outside play prior to commencing schoolwork, as it aids in focus. If you find your child needs this time to release his extra energy and refocus, simply structure it in right before homework time begins.

Ensure that there is a designated area for homework—either the kitchen table, dining room table, or a desk in a nearby quiet room. Your child's bedroom is *not* preferable, as there are far too many distractions. Additionally, you want to be close to your child to ensure that he is staying on task and to provide answers to any questions he may have.

If your child has a fair bit of homework, allow for small increments of time for each subject. For example, have him do thirty minutes of homework, and then give him a five-minute break that involves something simple, such as colouring, jumping on the trampoline, stretching, etc. Avoid television or video games at all costs.

Keep in mind that some children do homework best when it's quiet, some do better with a little background noise or music, and some kids work best with or without the short breaks. Find what works best for your child and go with it. You will find that the time will become far more productive and that there will be far less fighting or arguing.

Try to make the homework routine predictable and stress-free. Once the homework is done, check it over, and then help your child put the completed assignment in his homework folder and return all appropriate items to his backpack. No more hunting for it in the mornings or scrambling for lost papers.

Praise

Homework time is the perfect time to let your child know how well he's doing. Use this time to provide positive feedback for his hard work, and be sure to end each session on a positive note. It's important to remain relaxed and upbeat during homework time. Sometimes it's easy to focus on the negative, so be careful with your words. "That's not the way you're supposed to do that!" can be rephrased as, "I like how you did that, but let's try it this way!" Set up a reward system for the end of the week for an activity of your child's choice.

Note: If your child is in need of a tutor, find a tutor other than you to help. Look for one who would also be a good role model for your child. Boys with ADHD thrive with male tutors, and girls with ADHD thrive with female tutors. A tutor is a spectacular investment and also acts as a positive mentor in your child's life.

Bill of Rights for Children with ADHD

HELP ME TO FOCUS ...
Please teach me through my sense of touch.
I need "hands-on" and body movement.

I NEED TO KNOW WHAT COMES NEXT ...
Please give me a structured environment
where there is a dependable routine.
Give me an advance warning if there will be changes.

WAIT FOR ME, I'M STILL THINKING ...
Please allow me to go at my own pace.
If I'm rushed, I get confused and upset.

I'M STUCK, I CAN'T DO IT! ...
Please offer me options for problem solving.
If the road is blocked, I need to know the detours.

IS IT RIGHT? I NEED TO KNOW NOW ...
Please give me rich and immediate feedback
on how I'm doing.

I DIDN'T KNOW I WASN'T IN MY SEAT! ...
Please remind me to stop, think, and act.

AM I ALMOST DONE? ...
Please give me short work periods with short-term goals.

WHAT? ...
Please don't say, "I already told you that."
Tell me again, in different words.
Give me a signal. Draw me a symbol.

I KNOW IT'S ALL WRONG, ISN'T IT? ...
Please give me praise for partial success.
Reward me for self-improvement, not just for perfection.

BUT WHY DO I ALWAYS GET YELLED AT? ...
Please catch me doing something right
and praise me for the specific positive behaviour.
Remind me—and yourself—about my good points
when I'm having a bad day.

—Unknown

The biggest disability is a negative attitude!
—Unknown

THE IMPACT OF ADHD

It doesn't matter where you are; whether you're with your ADHD child at a movie theatre, a grocery store, a local playground, or your home, there are strategies for every situation. Below are the most important ones to consider.

ADHD in the Home
- Remember that your child's behaviour is related to a disorder. It is never intentional.

- Manage your own frustration and anger so that you can be in a position to help your child change daily patterns. In other words, look after yourself: Exercise, eat well, and do things you enjoy on your own, with your spouse, or with the entire family.

- Be patient with change and encourage baby steps with each change. Be sure to foster improvements and be calm about setbacks.

- Get help when you need it, either from your mate or from other caretakers, such as coaches, tutors, or babysitters.

- Make a list of the positive traits of your child and post them on the refrigerator. Look at this list often.

- Develop and repeat fun activities that allow your child to be at his best. Introduce new activities, and don't allow for frustration. Remind everyone involved that these activities are meant to be fun!

- Encourage athletic pursuits. Exercise does a world of good and has many, many benefits.
- Reinforce positive behaviour quickly, and follow through with negative consequences immediately.
- Expect only short periods of time when your child will be sitting still—usually, twenty-minute chunks at a time.
- Stand or sit close to your child and keep the list of instructions very short when giving direction. Remember, one thing at a time to start (baby steps).
- Be consistent.
- Provide structure.
- Be the advocate until your child can self-advocate. And even then, continue being an advocate.
- Believe in and support your child, always!

ADHD in Public

Children with ADHD can easily become overly stimulated and wild in public. They have a difficult time sitting still, they talk too loudly, they become bored easily, they ask a thousand questions, and they get into everything!

Here are some tips that should work at any given time:

- Try to anticipate the problems so that you can develop a plan of action. It is always better to act rather than to react.
- Ensure that your child understands the ground rules in advance, and let him know what the rewards and consequences will be for both compliance and noncompliance. *Follow through on consequences and rewards!* This is a must; otherwise, there is no reason to have ground rules in the first place.

- Be sure to identify an area that is private and to which you can take your child, if needed, to deal with any problems when you arrive at a public place. Examples of this would be the bathroom, your car, or simply a corner away from the public.

- Feel free to enlist the help of other adults if you attend a church or another place of worship. Don't feel as if you are alone. The benefit of religious groups is that they function as extended families.

- Safeguard a plan of structure that reduces any possibility that problems will occur. For example, if you know that your children will fight with each other relentlessly, keep them physically apart as best as you can. If you feel that this is not possible, then perhaps splurging for that last-minute sitter for one child will be well worth it.

- Do not let the problems of one child get in the way of everyone else's enjoyment. If at all possible, have a sitter on call, and entirely remove the child from the event without this significantly interfering with your involvement.

- Go back to the drawing board and come up with a better plan to address any repetition or recurrence if you can't figure out how to manage these problems properly the first time around. Many of these "public" problems do recur.

And if None of These Work . . .
- Say no in a calm, matter-of-fact tone.
- Set clear expectations with specific statements. The last thing you want to hear is, "You didn't say I couldn't touch my sister. You only said not to talk to her!"
- Put out an emotional fire.

- Give your child concrete jobs to do (for example, when you're at the grocery store, ask him to get twelve mushrooms, or anything that is easy on your list).

- Put energy into solving problems instead of adding fuel to an already growing fire.

The Impact of ADHD on Siblings

When a child or teen has ADHD, it affects everyone in the family: the child, parents, siblings, grandparents, etc. The specific focus on the child with ADHD can result in siblings feeling isolated, left out, and taken for granted. They may also receive less attention because of the principal needs of your child with ADHD. If the child's behaviour is disruptive, achieving a "normal" family life can become difficult. Siblings may feel the loss of peace and quiet, thus making them feel angry, guilty, resentful, or "lost." Additionally, stress that the parents are experiencing may be passed on to the rest of the family.

Due to the strong genetic component of ADHD, there is more of a chance that siblings will also have ADHD, a conduct disorder, or an emotional disorder. As we learn more about ADHD, there is still little information about the impact of chronic health conditions on a child's siblings. Various studies have found that siblings of children with a chronic illness are more likely to experience difficulties such as behaviour problems, shyness, substance abuse, lower self-esteem, poor peer relations resulting in difficulty making friends, loneliness, anger, anxiety, depression, or poor school grades. Note, though, that not all studies have found these negative effects. There is also some research suggesting that siblings are also likely to experience positive effects, such as greater compassion and positive peer relations over the long term.

Unfortunately, siblings of children with ADHD face a number of challenges in the home:

- Their needs often get less attention than those of the child with ADHD.
- They may be scolded more sharply when they err.
- Their successes may be less celebrated or taken for granted.
- They may be enlisted as assistant parents and then blamed if the sibling with ADHD misbehaves under their supervision.
- They may find their love for a brother or sister with ADHD mixed with jealousy and resentment.

Additionally, when a child or teen has ADHD, the needs of his siblings may get overlooked. Thus, siblings may experience a range of emotions, such as those listed here:

- anxiety over the ADHD sibling's behaviour
- anxiety over what other people think about the ADHD sibling's behaviour
- anxiety or worry over vacations or other changes in routine, because the ADHD sibling's symptoms will be less predictable
- resentment over the amount of time and attention the ADHD sibling receives
- worry about the disruption in family life the ADHD sibling creates
- sadness about being overlooked or about the lack of a "normal" family and childhood
- pride in their ability to help the ADHD sibling with his or her condition

How Children with ADHD and Their Siblings Interact

When the child with ADHD is younger than his sibling, the sibling may be expected to "babysit"—that is, supervise, play with, and protect the child with ADHD. But if the child with ADHD is older, younger siblings may imitate his behaviour. How siblings interact will partly depend on these factors:

- their ages in relation to each other
- their temperaments
- the quality of their relationships with their parents
- the quality of their relationships with each other
- the situation where parents favour one child over the other, or the children believe this is the case (the parents don't actually favour one or the other, but the children feel or think that they do)

When the child with ADHD also has oppositional defiant disorder or conduct disorder, he may be aggressive toward his sibling, as the sibling may seem like an "easy target." For this reason, it is important for parents to intervene in these situations earlier rather than later.

How to Help Siblings Cope

The very first, and, in my opinion, most significant step in coping is to learn about ADHD. Take the time to educate the entire family about ADHD. Instruct family members on how it affects their lives and on strategies to cope with living with an ADHDer. Talk about changes and adjustments that the family will need to make, and get everyone's input. It is extremely important to create an environment where siblings know it is acceptable to express their feelings and emotions.

Here are some specific ideas that you, as a parent, can use to help your other children cope:

- Try to maintain a reasonable, or "normal," family life to the best of your ability. Do this in spite of the disruption caused by ADHD. If needed, ask for suggestions from a psychiatrist, psychologist, counsellor, etc.—anyone who has been involved in the diagnosis of your ADHD child.

- Be consistent with daily routines and family routines. These are extremely important and helpful for the child with ADHD, and also important for the entire family. For example, have a schedule in a common area (e.g., the kitchen) so everyone is in the know as to who is where, who is picking whom up from school, who is going to practice, who is fixing dinner, etc.

- Keep in mind that just because one of your children has been diagnosed with ADHD, the same house rules for behaviour still apply to everyone at home, even more now than they did before the diagnosis. Rules and discipline should be *consistent* for the whole family.

- Ensure that your children keep up with sports or music lessons, playdates, tutoring, and other activities. Routine will be your best friend on many levels.

- Schedule special "family time" together, when the focus is on the entire family. The one afflicted with ADHD will be receiving individual focus at other times, so family time is essential.

- Remember that when you spend one-on-one time with your ADHD child, you must also spend some time alone with your other children on a regular basis. Siblings are often "rewarded" for being quiet and invisible, so because of this, they need special time with their parents too. This will give them the opportunity to express their feelings and emotions, which need to be taken seriously.

- Be there for all your children when they have questions or concerns. Explore their perceptions about ADHD, ask them what they wish to know, and listen to what they say. Their feelings are real and need to be heard and addressed in the same way as those of your child with ADHD.

- Involve siblings in a situation if they wish to be part of it. Let them help in the care of the child with ADHD or take on new responsibilities. Again, though, try to maintain the typical family roles. Older siblings can help, but they should not be expected to spend the bulk of their time taking care of their ADHD siblings. That's not their "job."

- Always recognize and reward siblings for their help. This is important. A little bit of help from them always goes a long way.

- Seek out ADHD organizations that have ADHD support groups if you feel siblings would benefit from these. They may benefit from meeting other siblings of children with ADHD.

- Be on the lookout for any other underlying sibling issues, such as depression or anxiety. Your other children may feel overwhelmed, so it's important that their feelings are being recognized and dealt with as well.

The Impact of ADHD on Parents

Now, of course, having a child with ADHD affects parents in many ways:

- The demands of a child with ADHD can be physically exhausting.

- The need to monitor the ADHD child's activities and actions can be psychologically exhausting.
- The ADHD child's inability to "listen" is frustrating.
- The ADHD child's behaviours, and your knowledge of their consequences, can make you anxious and stressed.
- Any basic differences between your personality and that of your child with ADHD can mean that you may find your child's behaviours especially difficult to accept.
- Frustration can lead to anger—and guilt over being angry—toward your ADHD child.

The key? Master compassion and consistency (i.e., love and structure)!

Parent Stress

Raising a child with ADHD can cause unhealthy amounts of stress in parents. Learning techniques to reduce stress can benefit both child and parent.

Food: Nourish yourself and eat well! By now, you should have made the decision to cook healthier for the family, so include yourself in this change—especially when you're on the go.

Exercise: Regular exercise increases chemicals in the brain that ease depression. In addition, the increased energy provided by exercise allows a parent to get more done. You will also be an excellent role model for your children. Remember that just twenty minutes of exercise increases the ability to focus immensely.

Sleep: This can be elusive and hard to come by, but find it! Your body, and your mind, will thank you in the morning!

Personal Appearance: A parent who feels good about his or her appearance gets a mental boost and the confidence to handle whatever challenges the ADHD child creates.

Make New Friends: Create a network of people who understand the difficulties of raising an ADHD child. Join an ADHD support group and meet parents of ADHD children—and ensure that your spouse is on board.

Time Management: This is crucial in getting important tasks done on a regular basis. Begin with the end goal in mind and create a simple daily schedule with easily attainable goals.

Be Present in the Moment: Concentrate on the way things look and feel *today*. Don't worry about yesterday, and don't worry about tomorrow. This will free your mind temporarily from the worries about past events and negative situations yet to come.

And remember: Stress management for parents of ADHD children is not a luxury. It is a necessity for the well-being of both child and parent.

SOME IMPORTANT EXTRA THINGS TO NOTE

- **Keep It Positive:** Because people with ADHD cannot put brakes on distractions, they will always attend to whatever is most appealing in their environment. Positive re-enforcement will get their attention, and constant criticism rarely improves a person's attitude, especially a person with ADHD. Children tend to remember the negative comments more than the positive ones, and it is the positive ones that you want emblazoned in their brains.

- **Keep It Calm:** No one (child or parent) can think clearly when stressed.

- **Keep It Organized:** Kids with ADHD often do their work and forget to hand it in the next morning. They need organizational support from parents *and* the school. This is where having an ADHD coach or tutor comes in handy.

- **Work with Your Child to Create a Plan:** Be aware of how ADHD can affect your child's strategy. Target each event—homework, sports, fun, or family time—and then work with your child to stay on track.

- **Maintain a Regular Schedule:** Work to consistently follow a plan with your child at home, at school, after school, and on weekends. Routine is *everything*!

- **Build a Support Team That Includes Parents, Teachers, Instructors, and Coaches:** Clearly communicate how ADHD affects your child's life. Discuss successes, and work together on the challenges. Also discuss disasters and meltdowns, and how they can be avoided.

- **Encourage Participation in After-School Activities:** Look for structured activities that use energy constructively and build social skills to achieve success in and out of school. These activities can be physical or mental. Either way, they are both extremely beneficial.

- **Ease the Strain of ADHD:** Keep routines fun and take breaks when times get tough to help relieve the stresses of ADHD.

- **Recognize Every Win:** Review your child's progress regularly and celebrate accomplishments, small and large. Even if your child did not do well on a test, let him know how proud of him you are for studying for it and being able to sit through the entire test. If he still doesn't seem happy because of the mark he received, reassure him that there will be more tests and that you can help him study more effectively for the next one.

- **Use Available Resources:** Take time to teach your child how to use calendars, organizers, and written reminders to help him stay focused in all parts of his day. Start small with these, as they too involve a learning process. Once your child has this mastered, it will become his "best friend."

- **Evaluate Your Child's Personal Strengths and Weaknesses:** Managing ADHD requires discipline, a positive attitude, and good planning skills. Again, the aid of a tutor who can mentor your child at the same time, or of an ADHD coach, is worth its weight in gold.

- **Understand the Challenges of ADHD:** Know that ADHD is a medical condition that makes it more difficult to control behaviour and attention. Be sure your child understands that it is not his fault that he has it. But, at the same time, ADHD is not an excuse either. Stress the importance of taking responsibility for recognizing and understanding the challenges of ADHD.

- **No Excuses:** Never allow your child or teen to say anything to the effect of, "I can't help it. I have ADHD." He *can* help it if he puts his mind to it.

THE FUTURE—WHAT WILL IT HOLD?

A child with ADHD will become a teenager with ADHD who will then, in turn, become an adult with ADHD. But just because your child has ADHD doesn't mean that his career opportunities aren't still wide open; they are just different.

If executive function is a severe problem, then chances are that finding the right career will pose a problem. However, below is a list of career fields that ADHDers absolutely thrive in:

Self-Employment: Once an ADHDer has found his passion, the world is his oyster. Owning his own business will give him a sense of satisfaction, as the rewards are huge and the independence he will feel is self-empowering. Owning a business will take some investment and gumption, but working a standard office job will usually make an ADHDer bored and cause him to lose his focus.

Medical Field (Doctor, Nurse, or Paramedic): You're probably thinking that there is no way someone with ADHD can sit through years of medical study, but many ADHDers find the field challenging and interesting enough to hold their attention. Additionally, the daily routine of a doctor, nurse, or paramedic changes regularly, so it grabs their interest continuously. An ADHDer's high energy, the variety of work this job field offers, and a good rapport with both patients and staff can all be bonuses in helping him succeed in this business.

Military: There are pros and cons for an ADHDer joining the military. On the pro side, entering the military requires only a high school diploma and passing a background check. Additionally, the field's rigid structure and the high energy and physical exertion it entails are also pluses. On the downside, some ADHDers may rebel against the strict discipline enforced. Moreover, in order to work their way up to becoming officers, they will require further education.

Law Enforcement (Firefighters and Police Officers): Most firefighters and police officers love their jobs, and there may be quite a bit of competition to find openings. However, if the ADHDer can get in, these types of occupations provide an excellent fit. ADHDers will thrive on the action and variety they are involved in daily, as well as on relying on their own skills and judgments. The only disadvantages are that during downtimes there are periods of mundane paperwork and boredom, in addition to the need to deal with authority figures.

Sales: Having freedom is huge for an ADHDer, which is where being a high-level, independent salesperson comes into play, especially a commission salesperson. Even though this does require a college education and good people skills, a determined ADHDer can attain them both. This results in an ADHDer enjoying the liberty to make his own schedule, work autonomously, and create a system in which he can work at his own pace rather than at one that is dictated. It helps an ADHDer develop his self-confidence and work on core issues such as organization and multitasking.

Overall, finding the right career for anyone is difficult, and even more so for someone with ADHD. As long as an ADHDer seeks something that offers creativity, independence, and variety, he can't go wrong. The last two years of high school are key, and working with an academic counsellor is important, as this figure will be able to help the ADHDer find a focus—a focus that he loves and is passionate about. This will, at the very least, get him started on the path to finding the right direction to avoid becoming lost in a sea of uncertainty.

Why fit in when you were born to stand out?
—Dr. Seuss

QUICK FACTS ABOUT ADHD THAT EVERY PARENT SHOULD KNOW

- In a classroom with thirty students, there will be between one and three children who have some form of ADHD.
- Boys are diagnosed with ADHD three times more often than girls.
- Emotional development in children with ADHD is 30 percent slower than in their non-ADHD peers. This means that a child who is ten years old will have the emotional development of a seven-year-old, and a twenty-year-old will have the emotional maturity of a fourteen-year-old.
- One fourth of children with ADHD have serious learning disabilities, such as difficulties with oral expression, listening skills, reading comprehension, and/or math.
- Sixty-five percent of children with ADHD exhibit problems with defiance or problems with authority figures. This can include demonstrating verbal hostility and temper tantrums.
- Seventy-five percent of boys diagnosed with ADHD have hyperactivity.
- Sixty percent of girls diagnosed with ADHD have hyperactivity.
- Fifty percent of children with ADHD experience sleep

problems. This is without the use of medication. If they are using medication, the percentage is higher by approximately 20 percent.

- Teenagers with ADHD are four times more likely to get traffic citations than non-ADHD drivers. They have four times as many car accidents and are seven times more likely to have a second accident.

- Twenty-one percent of teenagers with ADHD skip school on a regular basis, and 35 percent drop out of school before finishing high school.

- Forty-five percent of children with ADHD have been suspended from school at least once.

- Thirty percent of children with ADHD have had to repeat a year in school.

- Teenagers with ADHD are more likely to turn to street drugs than non-ADHD teenagers.

- ADHD teens are also more likely to get into trouble with the law on more than one occasion during their lives.

So now you're wondering whether having ADHD is a good thing or a bad thing. Well, it's still very much a good thing. It is very important to keep the above facts in mind so that they never become options for your child. When reading these statistics, it is very easy to focus on all the negatives and problems associated with ADHD. But there is an amazing slew of positives that outnumber the negatives immensely. For every one negative, there are *at least* three positives. Just see below and you'll know what I mean!

The Hidden Gifts of ADHD

So with all this being said, you're probably now thinking, "What are the so-called 'hidden gifts' of ADHD?" Here are just a few traits that are more prevalent in people with ADHD. Not everyone with ADHD has all of these characteristics, and yes, you don't have to have ADHD to possess them. But ADHDers have these qualities and mannerisms even more so, and this is why we love them immensely.

- adaptable
- athletic
- charismatic
- charming
- compassionate
- creative in many, many ways
- difficult to fool
- doesn't harbor resentment
- down-to-earth
- dreamer
- driven
- eager for acceptance and willing to work for it
- empathetic toward the feelings of others
- energetic

- enthusiastic
- fast-thinking
- feels things deeply
- flexible
- forgives mistakes easily
- fun
- fun-loving
- good judge of character
- great at finding lost items
- hardworking
- humble
- humourous
- hyper-focused
- idea generator
- imaginative
- innovative
- intense when interested in something or someone
- inquisitive
- insightful
- intuitive
- inventive
- less likely to get in a rut
- looks past the surface appearance to the core of people, situations, and issues
- loyal
- mechanically inclined
- more likely to do things out of want rather than out of necessity

- multi-talented
- not secretive
- observant
- open-minded
- optimistic
- original
- outgoing
- passionate
- perceptively acute
- personable
- problem-solving ability
- quick at doing engaging, interesting, enjoyable activities
- quick to grasp essentials
- resilient
- resourceful
- responsive to positive reinforcement
- risk-taking
- sees unique relationships between people and things
- sees things from a unique perspective
- sensitive
- spontaneous
- tenacious
- trusting
- visual
- visionary
- warmhearted
- wholehearted when making an effort

I encourage everyone who has ADHD, or knows someone who has ADHD, to cut out a copy of this list (see Appendix) and keep it handy for those times you forget what a blessing having ADHD can be.

ADHD AND FAME

When you mention ADHD to a child who *has* ADHD, many feelings surface, such as loneliness, frustration, anger, and confusion. This primarily stems from the child's lack of education on ADHD, because no one has really taken the time to sit down with him to explain it and answer his questions. Additionally, and most importantly, his self-esteem is at an all-time low. Ensuring that the child understands his condition is imperative. This will allow him to learn to live with it and advocate for himself when you're not around. Your child's self-esteem is shaped not only by how he thinks about himself and by what he expects of himself, but also by how other people think and feel about him.

The more children with ADHD know, the better off they are. We all know that knowledge is power. So let's start the learning—and teaching—process when they are young to ensure that they know they're not alone, and that even some of the most brilliant minds in the world, both past and present, lived or currently live with ADHD as well. Here are some examples, just to name a few:

Albert Einstein
Ansel Adams
Babe Ruth
Bill Gates
Britney Spears
Bruce Jenner
Channing Tatum
Christopher Knight
Courtney Love
Howie Mandel
James Carville
Jamie Oliver
Jason Earles
Jennifer Connelly
Jim Carrey
John F. Kennedy
Justin Timberlake
Karina Smirnoff
Kurt Cobain
Liv Tyler
Magic Johnson
Malcolm Forbes
Melissa Joan Hart
Michael Phelps
Michelle Rodriguez
Napolean

Daniel Bedingfield
David Neeleman
Ernest Hemingway
Edgar Allan Poe
Emma Watson
Forrest Griffin
Glenn Beck
Heather Kuzmich
Hilary Duff
Norman Schwarzkopf
Paul Orfalea
Paris Hilton
Pete Rose
Richard Branson
Robert Frost
Robin Williams
Roxy Olin
Salma Hayek
Solange Knowles
Ted Turner
Terry Bradshaw
Ty Pennington
Whoopi Goldberg
Will Smith
Zooey Deschanel

This list could go on and on, but it's just a snippet to show you that some of the greatest minds in the world have ADHD too...which is probably why they are considered some of the greatest minds!

RESOURCES

So you happen to be in a unique situation that I haven't mentioned, and you have no idea what to do. What do you do? Where do you turn? Chances are, you head straight for the Internet, but how do you know if the websites you're looking at are reliable? Here's a list of five key factors you should look out for:

1. Look for sites that are already established and have been around for some time.

2. Look for sites with expertise. Make sure that related articles and posts are from specialists in the kinds of information you are seeking.

3. Check the date. Be sure that the articles that are posted present the most up-to-date information available. Studies happen continuously, so findings change regularly. One way to check for this is to look for a "last updated" date on the page or the site.

4. Look at the way the website appears. If a site looks poorly designed and amateurish, then chances are it was created by amateurs. But be careful—just because a website is professionally designed doesn't mean it's reliable.

5. Consider these questions if you're not sure whether to trust a website:

    • *Are you visiting a secure site? (Does your antivirus program tell you that it's not safe?)*

- *Does the website ask you for personal information?*
- *Does the website continuously send you to other links that are unrelated to what you are seeking in the first place?*
- *Is there a slew of advertisements for items that are unrelated to what you initially went on the website to research?*
- *Is there contact information, such as a phone number or e-mail address?*
- *Does the site offer inappropriate content, such as pornography or illegal materials? (For example, does the site have a link to another site where you can buy Adderall or Ritalin online?)*
- *Does the website ask for a credit card to verify identity or for personal information that does not seem necessary to disclose?*

Here are a few of my favourite sites:

CADDAC – Centre for ADHD Awareness, Canada
www.caddac.ca

CHADD – Children and Adults with Attention Deficit Hyperactivity Disorder
www.chadd.org

ADDitude Magazine
www.additudemag.com

ADHD Aware
www.adhdaware.org

National Resource Center on ADHD
www.help4adhd.org

ADD Resources
www.addresources.org

CADDRA – Canadian ADHD Resource Alliance
www.caddra.ca

CCHR – Citizens Commission on Human Rights
www.cchrint.org
The ADDvocates
www.theaddvocates.com

CONCLUSION

It's simple. For the most part, ADHD is something someone is born with. There is no cure for it, so you need to find a way for your child to be able to live with it effectively. In doing so, you must look for ways in which ADHD becomes complementary to his lifestyle rather than detrimental to it. This can be hard on so many levels, especially for a young child or teenager, but also for adults who struggle with it.

Outsiders have no idea why your child is like this, so they come up with their own conclusions, which are usually incorrect. Teachers and coaches constantly want to label your child to the point where he is suddenly in a class for "troubled students." And his doctor or therapist wants to medicate him to the point where your child actually *believes* that there *is* something wrong with him. So what do you do?

Educate: This applies not only to yourself but also to other people who are involved in your child's life. Give these people strategies that you know will work. And don't forget to educate your child too, because he knows himself best. The more he knows about ADHD, the better he can live with it.

Advocate: Let people know that, "No, you will not medicate!" because you don't want your child to become one of the statistics of children who end up with severe complications from medication. And teach your child to advocate for himself, because when you're not around, he'll need his inner strength to come through.

Nourish: Feed your child and feed him well. Cultivate proper eating habits and instill a suitable vitamin or supplement regimen that complements his current lifestyle. Remember, monkey see, monkey do—if your child sees you eating well and taking your vitamins, he too will be more inclined to hop on board.

Set routines: When he knows what to expect, this will make your ADHD child's life so much easier. And, in turn, it will make your life easier as well. Routinely provide security, rhythm, and harmony, and ease the stress of everyday life.

And never, ever forget to exercise constant patience and love. Patience is a virtue that can be cultivated and nurtured over time. Add love and you will be pleasantly surprised by how relaxing and peaceful the quality of your life, and especially that of your ADHD child, will become.

Be who you are and say what you feel,
because those who mind don't matter
and those who matter don't mind.
—Dr. Seuss

APPENDIX

Template Letter to the Teacher

Bill of Rights for Children with ADHD

Hidden Gifts of ADHD

Famous People with ADHD

Sample Weekly Menu Plan

Supplements and Their Best Food Sources

Organic and Inorganic Foods—What
to Buy and What Not to Buy

List of Resources

List of Food Dyes and Additives

Template Letter to the Teacher

To Jonathan's Teachers:

Jonathan Smith will be in your class this year. Over the years, we have found it helpful to give teachers some background about him, in addition to the IEP in his file. This often ensures a successful beginning to the school year.

Jon has Attention Deficit Hyperactivity Disorder (ADHD). He is not on medication for various reasons and we have no plans to put him on any medication in the near future. Jon has a great sense of humour, and tapping into this early in the year usually works well. Jon takes criticism personally and hates being yelled at. He won't always let you know it, but he worries and is very sensitive. He might act cool and tough, but if he has had a bad day, he falls apart when he gets home.

Jon is excited about the new year. He wants to settle down and "be mature and responsible." He says this at the beginning of every year, but he can't always succeed. The last school year was a difficult one, and Jon's self-esteem is pretty beaten up.

We have attached a list of things that have worked in some situations.

We welcome any ideas you have to keep Jon engaged in school while boosting his self-esteem and helping him succeed. Please contact us at any time by phone or by e-mail. We have flexible schedules and are able to meet whenever it is convenient for you. We look forward to working with you in the upcoming year.

Sincerely,
Jonathan's Parents

Bill of Rights for Children with ADHD

HELP ME TO FOCUS ...
Please teach me through my sense of touch.
I need "hands-on" and body movement.

I NEED TO KNOW WHAT COMES NEXT ...
Please give me a structured environment
where there is a dependable routine.
Give me an advance warning if there will be changes.

WAIT FOR ME, I'M STILL THINKING ...
Please allow me to go at my own pace.
If I'm rushed, I get confused and upset.

I'M STUCK, I CAN'T DO IT! ...
Please offer me options for problem solving.
If the road is blocked, I need to know the detours.

IS IT RIGHT? I NEED TO KNOW NOW ...
Please give me rich and immediate feedback
on how I'm doing.

I DIDN'T KNOW I WASN'T IN MY SEAT! ...
Please remind me to stop, think, and act.

AM I ALMOST DONE? ...
Please give me short work periods with short-term goals.

WHAT? ...
Please don't say, "I already told you that."
Tell me again, in different words.
Give me a signal. Draw me a symbol.

I KNOW IT'S ALL WRONG, ISN'T IT? ...
Please give me praise for partial success.
Reward me for self-improvement, not just for perfection.

BUT WHY DO I ALWAYS GET YELLED AT? ...
Please catch me doing something right
and praise me for the specific positive behaviour.
Remind me—and yourself—about my good points
when I'm having a bad day.

—Unknown

Hidden Gifts of ADHD

- adaptable
- athletic
- charismatic
- charming
- compassionate
- creative in many, many ways
- difficult to fool
- doesn't harbor resentment
- down-to-earth
- dreamer
- driven
- eager for acceptance and willing to work for it
- empathetic toward the feelings of others
- energetic
- enthusiastic
- fast-thinking
- feels things deeply
- flexible
- forgives mistakes easily
- fun
- fun-loving
- good judge of character
- great at finding lost items
- hardworking

- humble
- humourous
- hyper-focused
- idea generator
- imaginative
- innovative
- intense when interested in something or someone
- inquisitive
- insightful
- intuitive
- inventive
- less likely to get in a rut
- looks past the surface appearance to the core of people, situations, and issues
- loyal
- mechanically inclined
- more likely to do things out of want than out of necessity
- multi-talented
- not secretive
- observant
- open-minded
- optimistic
- original
- outgoing
- passionate
- perceptively acute
- personable
- problem-solving ability
- quick at doing engaging, interesting, enjoyable activities

- quick to grasp essentials
- resilient
- resourceful
- responsive to positive reinforcement
- risk-taking
- sees unique relationships between people and things
- sees things from a unique perspective
- sensitive
- spontaneous
- tenacious
- trusting
- visual
- visionary
- warmhearted
- wholehearted when making an effort

Famous People with ADHD

Albert Einstein	Justin Timberlake
Ansel Adams	Karina Smirnoff
Babe Ruth	Kurt Cobain
Bill Gates	Liv Tyler
Britney Spears	Magic Johnson
Bruce Jenner	Malcolm Forbes
Channing Tatum	Melissa Joan Hart
Christopher Knight	Michael Phelps
Courtney Love	Michelle Rodriguez
Daniel Bedingfield	Napolean
David Neeleman	Norman Schwarzkopf
Ernest Hemingway	Paul Orfalea
Edgar Allan Poe	Paris Hilton
Emma Watson	Pete Rose
Forrest Griffin	Richard Branson
Glenn Beck	Robert Frost
Heather Kuzmich	Robin Williams
Hilary Duff	Roxy Olin
Howie Mandel	Salma Hayek
James Carville	Solange Knowles
Jamie Oliver	Ted Turner
Jason Earles	Terry Bradshaw
Jennifer Connelly	Ty Pennington
Jim Carrey	Whoopi Goldberg
John F. Kennedy	Will Smith
	Zooey Deschanel

Sample Weekly Menu Plan

	Monday	Tuesday	Wednesday	Thursday	Friday	Saturday	Sunday
Breakfast	Whole-grain toast with nut butter Fresh fruit Organic milk	Granola with organic milk Fresh fruit	Plain oatmeal with fresh berries and nuts Fresh fruit	Toasted whole-grain bagel (half) with cream cheese Small smoothie with protein powder	Granola with organic milk Fresh fruit	Whole-grain toast with nut butter Fresh fruit Organic milk	2 egg omelet with sautéed veggies and cheese Whole-grain toast Fresh fruit
Lunch	Dijon turkey wrap Small coleslaw Fresh fruit	Spinach salad with several mixed veggies Whole-grain roll Fresh fruit	Lean roast beef and veggie stuffed pita Fresh fruit	Egg salad sandwich on whole-grain bread Small green salad Fresh fruit	2 slices thin crust pizza Small green salad Fresh fruit	Tuna wrap with fresh veggies Small green salad Fresh fruit	Caesar salad Small whole-grain roll Fresh fruit
Dinner	Oven roasted salmon Roasted rosemary nugget potatoes Steamed veggies of your choice	Chicken and veggie stir-fry with brown rice or rice noodles	BBQ pork chops Garlic mashed potatoes Steamed veggies of your choice	Chicken quesadilla Brown rice with mixed veggies	Striploin steak Baked potato Steamed veggies of your choice	Spaghetti and meatballs Green salad (with several mixed fresh veggies)	Roast turkey breast Mashed potatoes Steamed veggies of your choice

Supplements and Their Best Food Sources

Thiamine

tuna	pecans
beans	brown rice
fortified cereals	asparagus
Brussels sprouts	kale
sunflower seeds	potatoes
pork chops	eggs
pistachios	liver (beef, pork, chicken)
macadamia nuts	marmite (yeast extract)

Niacin (Vitamin B3)

wheat bran	peanuts
pork chops	fortified cereals
chicken	marmite (yeast extract)
tuna	liver
salmon	paprika
mackerel	sun-dried tomatoes
trout	mushrooms
herring	potatoes
sardines	cottage cheese
beef	

Pyridoxine (Vitamin B6)

wheat bran	pistachios
raw garlic	sesame seeds
liver	pork
tuna	molasses
salmon	hazelnuts
mackerel	potatoes
cod	sweet potatoes
halibut	carrots
trout	avocados
sunflower seeds	soy beverages

Magnesium

spinach
potatoes
okra
fortified cereals
soy beverages
tofu
sunflower seeds
hummus
almonds

cashews
pine nuts
flaxseeds
peanuts
salmon
halibut
mackerel
pollack
crab

Calcium

spinach
kale
turnip greens
milk products
cheese
tofu
almonds

yogurt
salmon
mackerel
sardines
anchovies
molasses

Zinc

wheat germ
fortified cereals
milk
cheese
yogurt
liver
beef
veal
lamb
turkey
pork
chicken
baked beans

pine nuts
peanuts
cashews
almonds
lentils
eggs
oysters
scallops
lobster
clams
mussels
anchovies
shrimp

Iron

clams	almonds
oysters	beef
liver	lamb
squash	beans
pumpkin seeds	whole-grains
cashews	spinach
hazelnuts	Swiss chard
peanuts	tofu
dark chocolate	

Omega-3

wheat germ	mussels
squash	oysters
radishes	salmon
edamame	sardines
fortified milk and yogurt	trout
eggs	tuna
anchovies	snapper
caviar	beans
clams	pecans
cod	flaxseeds
mackerel	walnuts
lobster	almonds
halibut	

Organic and Inorganic Foods—What to Buy and What Not to Buy

Buy Organic	Don't Buy Organic
potatoes	onions
peanut butter	bananas
milk	pineapples
apples	avocados
meat	cabbage
nectarines	asparagus
spinach	mangoes
peaches	kiwis
pears	cantaloupe
strawberries	watermelons
bell peppers	sweet potatoes
eggs	mushrooms
grapes	honey
dairy products	grapefruit

Note: Organic foods tend to go bad much faster than inorganic foods, so be sure either to purchase small quantities of them or eat them quickly. Additionally, organic foods will also have more bacteria a week after purchase, as organic farmers are usually less efficient in getting their products to the market.

- If there are only **four numbers** in the PLU code, this indicates that the item was grown **conventionally** with the use of pesticides.

- If there are **five numbers** in the PLU code, and the number starts with "**8**," this tells you that the item is a **genetically modified** fruit or vegetable.

- If there are **five numbers** in the PLU code, and the number starts with "**9**," this tells you that the item was grown **organically**.

CADDAC – Centre for ADHD Awareness, Canada
www.caddac.ca

CHADD – Children and Adults with Attention Deficit Hyperactivity Disorder
www.chadd.org

ADDitude Magazine
www.additudemag.com

ADHD Aware
www.adhdaware.org

National Resource Center on ADHD
www.help4adhd.org

ADD Resources
www.addresources.org

CADDRA – Canadian ADHD Resource Alliance
www.caddra.ca

CCHR – Citizens Commission on Human Rights
www.cchrint.org

The ADDvocates
www.theaddvocates.com

List of Food Dyes and Additives

Sodium Benzoate (food preservative): commonly used in fruit pies, jams, beverages, salads, relishes, and sauerkraut

Blue No. 1 (Brilliant Blue): commonly used in some Yoplait products, some Jell-O dessert products, Fruity Cheerios, Froot Loops, some Pop-Tarts products, some Oscar Mayer Lunchables, Duncan Hines Whipped Chocolate Frosting, Skittles candy, Jolly Rancher Screaming Sours Soft & Chewy Candy, Eclipse gum, and Fanta grape soda

Blue No. 2 (Indigotine): commonly used in Froot Loops, Pop-Tarts products, Duncan Hines Moist Deluxe Strawberry Supreme Premium Cake Mix, Betty Crocker Rich & Creamy Cherry Frosting, M&M's milk chocolate candy, M&M's milk chocolate peanut candy, and Wonka Nerds grape and strawberry flavoured candy

Green No. 3: rarely used, but can still be found in some candy, beverages, ice creams, and puddings

Orange B: rarely used, but can still be found in some sausage casings

Red No. 3 (Carmoisine): found in some candy, cake icing, and chewing gum

Red No. 40 (Allura Red): by far the most popular and commonly used in some Yoplait products, some Jello-O dessert products, Quaker Instant Oatmeal, Froot Loops, Trix, some Pop-Tarts products, Oscar Mayer Lunchables, Hostess Twinkies, some Pillsbury rolls and frostings, some Betty Crocker and Duncan Hines frostings, and more

Yellow No. 5 (Tartrazine): commonly used in Nabisco Cheese Nips Four Cheese crackers, Hunt's Snack Pack Pudding products, Lucky Charms, Eggo waffle and other waffle products, some Pop-Tarts products, various Kraft macaroni-and-cheese products, Betty Crocker products, Hamburger Helper products, and more (This food dye has been tested alone and has a direct link to hyperactivity.)

Yellow No. 6 (Sunset Yellow): commonly used in Betty Crocker Fruit Roll-Ups, some Jell-O dessert products and instant puddings, Fruity Cheerios, Trix, some Eggo waffle products, some Kraft macaroni-and-cheese products, Betty Crocker frostings, some M&M's and Skittles candy, Sunkist orange soda, and Fanta orange soda

ABOUT THE AUTHOR

Karen Ryan is a seasoned nutritionist as well as an ADHD coach and behaviour interventionist for school-aged children and teens. She is a firm believer in the correlation between food and mood and that a clean diet is the best medicine for sound health of body and mind. Guided by her extensive education, research, and experience in clinical and holistic nutrition, Karen dedicates her focus to helping all people, especially children and teens with ADHD, eat healthier and live happier.

As an active member of several organizations, Karen also devotes her time to working on behalf of Children and Adults Against Drugging America (CHAADA), the Citizens Commission on Human Rights (CCHR), the Canadian Society of Nutrition Management (CSNM), the Pacific Society of Nutrition Management (PSNM), and the Canadian Association of Natural Nutritional Practitioners (CANNP). In addition, Karen is the founder of The ADDvocates, an organization aimed at raising awareness of ADHD.

She currently resides in Vancouver, BC, with her husband and two children. Karen counts her vivacious son, who was diagnosed with ADHD at age seven, as her greatest inspiration for writing this book.

CPSIA information can be obtained at www.ICGtesting.com
Printed in the USA
BVOW04s2157290914

368555BV00006B/3/P